Emotional Release Therapy

Also by Walter Weston

Pray Well: A Holistic Guide to Health and Renewal

Healing Others: A Practical Guide

Healing Yourself: A Practical Guide

How Prayer Heals: A Scientific Approach

Emotional Release Therapy

WALTER WESTON

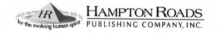

HAMPTON ROADS
PUBLISHING COMPANY, INC.

Hampton Roads Publishing Company, Inc.
1125 Stoney Ridge Road
Charlottesville, VA 22902

434-296-2772
fax: 434-296-5096
e-mail: hrpc@hrpub.com
www.hrpub.com

If you are unable to order this book from your local
bookseller, you may order directly from the publisher.
Call 1-800-766-8009, toll-free.

Library of Congress Cataloging-in-Publication Data

Weston, Walter.
  Emotional release therapy : healing life's painful emotions / Walter
Weston.
    p. cm.
  Summary: "Introduces a simple technique that permanently removes painful and
traumatic memories along with self-destructive emotional states like depression, grief,
fear, and anger. Since emotional pain is often the root cause of many physical
diseases, ERT can likewise alleviate painful conditions and speed recovery from
disease"--Provided by publisher.
  ISBN 1-57174-435-5 (alk. paper)
  1. Emotions. 2. Psychotherapy. I. Title.
  RC489.E45W47 2005
  616.89'14--dc22
                          2005025916

ISBN 1-57174-435-5
10 9 8 7 6 5 4 3 2
Printed on acid-free paper in the United States

Contents

Foreword

Perhaps Emotional Release Therapy could only have been developed by a man who is both a healer and an ordained minister. It is a sort of blend of energy medicine and prayer—with some silent psychotherapy thrown in! It is the simplest, most powerful technique I know of, requiring neither elaborate equipment nor extensive training.

You can heal yourself, and you can help others heal themselves. You can even heal animals. What is most remarkable, you can help people heal deep emotional traumas without their having to say a word—which means you can help people heal from traumas that are so painful that they cannot bear even to speak about them.

It sounds like magic. Can it be true?

Yes, it can.

So where does the magic come from? It doesn't come from the head. It comes from the heart. It is the heart that connects us with the force that heals.

You might ask whether this fruit of Walter Weston's work is science, or medicine, or religion. But maybe it isn't important to decide. Maybe, in fact, it is almost a meaningless question. Maybe our civilization has constructed too many barriers between three ways of approaching the same reality. Maybe it is time to tear down some of those barriers and reconnect with the real magic that is available to all who know how to come from the heart—and all who can learn to do so.

Do you believe in the power of prayer?

If not, you are behind the times.

Do you believe that you yourself can heal your physical, emotional, and spiritual traumas?

If not, you are behind the times.

Do you believe that you can help others heal?

If not, you are behind the times.

Here's the book that will help you experience a deeper, more hopeful reality. It only requires that you be willing to try it, as I have.

—Frank DeMarco, chairman, Hampton Roads Publishing

Introduction

Emotional Release Therapy may be one of the most important books you will ever read. Its impact on people could mark a turning point in human history as human emotional pain is conquered in all people in all the nations of the world. *Emotional Release Therapy* will teach you how to remove all your emotional pain as well as the emotional pain of others. Do you know the implications of this?

Adults can have every painful hurt removed; battered women, crime victims, auto accident victims, veterans with post-traumatic stress disorder, and everyone in the world can have painful memories removed. People suffering from destructive emotional states like depression, grief, fear, anger, and anxiety will be normal in a few hours. There will be little need for psychotherapy or medications.

Emotionally and physically traumatized children—battered children—can become healthy and whole as if the trauma had never happened. Children and youth whose emotional pain has been removed by ERT see wondrous results. It enables them to live up to their potential. It causes them to behave responsibly. It may help juvenile delinquents behave normally. It may raise the IQ of infants. It may reduce the onset of genetic diseases. Many diseases have psychosomatic causes. Removing emotional pain can cure or alleviate the diseases of many persons.

Emotional Release Therapy

All this is done with Emotional Release Therapy (ERT), an entirely new approach to healing your emotional pain. Everything you need to practice Emotional Release Therapy (ERT) is covered in this book.

Emotional Release Therapy removes all of your emotional pain within hours. Imagine releasing the emotional trauma of every painful memory you've ever had! Imagine permanently removing all negative emotional states! Imagine helping others do the same! I know this sounds too wonderful to be true. I was amazed when I first discovered how simple and easy it is to use Emotional Release Therapy (ERT).

Discovering ERT

It's amazing how I found the basis for ERT. In February 1994, I went to Montreal to visit a medical clairvoyant who had promised to teach me how to read energy fields. She had an office where medical doctors sent patients whom they could not diagnose. She could.

She had her own agenda and I found myself healing patients at ten- to 15-minute intervals, when I usually take an hour with a patient. During this time, I met the most depressed woman I have ever seen, using a walker to hobble around. Diane had been in an auto accident ten years before and been injured so badly that she couldn't teach anymore. I had only ten minutes to work with her and regretted that I didn't have more time. I gave her written instructions for healing herself.

A month later, Diane phoned me. She told me that all her injuries had been healed and she was free of pain. Then she made a request. She said, "The next time you are in Montreal, would you heal my depression?"

I didn't know how to heal depression, but I gave her an easy yes because I never expected to be in Montreal again. But in May, three months later, I was in Montreal once again, registering at a healing conference. And who should be seated near the registration table but Diane.

She gave me a big hug and said, "I knew you'd be here. Now you can heal my depression."

I said, "Let's meet tomorrow at noon." I didn't have clue as to how to take her depression away. But I am very intuitive. That evening I prayed that God would provide me the answer in a dream. I awoke the next morning with nothing. I was getting nervous.

I went to the conference and at 10 A.M. the speaker, an Indiana psychologist named Cher Wendt, provided me with God's answer to relieving depression. Dr. Wendt spoke a sentence or two about her technique, Radiant Heart Therapy. It was enough to spark my creative flow.

At noon, I met with Diane in a psychologist's office. I placed my flattened hand just above her heart, told her to place a color in her heart, and then to release the feelings of depression into the color. My hand felt her release as heat. She released for 40 minutes and reported, "Oh, I feel so light." Her depression was completely gone. I was shocked at how easy it had been. I also realized the potential of this simple technique.

This was the beginning of Emotional Release Therapy. I talked with Cher Wendt several times after that and then we went our separate ways.

A New Approach Was Needed

In the past century of clinical research and experience, medications and psychotherapy have not discovered a way to remove emotional pain. They mask it, but it is still there.

This being true, it becomes obvious that these two approaches have reached a dead end. Their assumptions about the nature, cause, and cure of emotional pain must be faulty. Therefore, a new understanding and approach are needed.

That is what this book offers, an entirely new understanding and approach. Here we take a quantum leap forward to a new understanding that, once grasped, makes sense. We're talking about a whole new field of understanding that so simplifies treatment that it sounds far too easy to be true.

Throughout human history, painful memories and destructive emotional states have plagued humanity. They can haunt us, steal our happiness, hamper our living. They can contribute to our ill health. They can kill us! We can become obsessed by emotional pain. It is like being possessed by something that will never let us go.

ERT Is Easy to Learn and Apply

You can learn to practice the basic skills of Emotional Release Therapy in a few hours. ERT can be practiced with people of all ages, including infants. It can be practiced on emotionally traumatized animals, like dogs, cats, and horses.

In the past 11 years, I have practiced ERT with more than four hundred people. I have used this experience as the basis for teaching more than three thousand people in the United States, Canada, India, and South Africa, in 12-hour workshops, to practice Emotional Release Therapy with competence. You will read these people's stories throughout this book.

Like many people, my motto is "If it works, use it." The practical truth of what I write in this book is evident in the outcomes that you will produce. Everyone who has practiced Emotional Release Therapy knows that it works and that it works for everyone, producing consistent and predictable results.

The symptoms of those diseases with a strong emotional element in them are alleviated or cured by Emotional Release Therapy. I have witnessed some cancer patients whose symptoms have been alleviated.

Empathy Developed by Emotional Release Therapy

ERT opens people to feeling empathy and thus displaying compassion for the emotional pain of others. Compassionate men would make the women and children in these men's lives extremely happy. In this way, ERT could prevent millions of divorces.

People Opened to God

After ERT, people are opened to an awareness of God. Most men have never experienced God. ERT could enable millions of men to have this experience.

It Will Change Your Life Forever

Do you know what else will happen when you have released all your emotional pain? It will change your life forever.

Emotional pain masks who you really are. Emotional pain has shaped your attitudes, thoughts, beliefs, actions, personality, relationships, and lifestyle. Your destructive emotions enslave you.

Emotional pain produces a destructive energy that blocks you from learning and growing and from achieving personal and vocational success. Through releasing that pain, you may acquire the happiness and satisfaction you have long sought.

Your memory may improve. You may become more intelligent. You may clearly feel the emotional pain of others and respond to their needs with compassion. You may become more loving and understanding. You may experience God more intensely. Your physical health may dramatically improve.

These are the wonders of Emotional Release Therapy.

Part I

A New Mode of Healing

1

The Heart of the Matter

My joy is gone, grief is upon me, my heart is sick.

—Jer. 8:18

My heart is broken and heavy, and I cannot fight back the tears.

—An abandoned wife

Where in the brain could we possibly store our emotions? I have never felt fear or anger or sadness in my brain circuits. I have never felt any emotions in my brain. How about you? If emotional pain were stored in the brain, then you could think it away. But you can't. This seems obvious!

Since childhood, you have known where most of your emotions are stored. Where do you feel your joy, your love, your lightness, your happiness? Where do you experience your loneliness, anger, sadness, worry, and fear? In your heart, naturally. We have all felt our hearts filled with love and joy and, at other times, with emotional pain and heaviness.

For thousands of years, long before the birth of psychotherapy and modern medications, poets, seers, saints, lovers, and the common person knew where we store our emotions. They have told us in countless ways that we store our emotions in our hearts.

The ancient truth came to us more than 2,500 years ago as the Psalmists wrote about heartfelt states:

- "How long must I have sorrow in my heart all day long?" (Ps. 13:2).

- "My heart is in anguish within me, the terrors of death have fallen upon me" (Ps. 55:4).

- "Insults have broken my heart, so that I am in despair" (Ps. 69:20).

- "With my whole heart I cry" (Ps. 119:145).

What does this imply? Where does this point? Since our emotions are located in the heart, the obvious truth is that we store our emotions in our hearts.

The next logical step is to conclude that each of us likely stores our whole emotional history in the heart. This includes our cherished emotions like love, joy, and peace, as well as our destructive emotions like fear, sadness, and anger.

Like books in a library, the emotions in the heart are stored in separate areas. In one area we store our anger, in another our fears, in another our happiness, in another our joys, and on and on. These emotional storage areas begin forming in infancy, with each area enlarging as we experience more and more of the specific emotion stored in that area.

For instance, the first fear may begin to be stored before birth while we are in our mother's womb, or at birth. Throughout a lifetime, that fear area can grow in size. Or it can be diminished by experiencing constructive emotions like love, confidence, and security.

If we go back in time to the first fear and remove it, which is possible to do with ERT, we remove all fear, because the storage area created by the first fear has been removed.

Once we accept these obvious truths, we naturally ask the question: How can I remove the destructive emotions from my heart? How can I rid

4

myself of my fears, my sadness, my anger, my emotional pain? The answer is: through the new process of Emotional Release Therapy. The second question we should ask is, how can I intensify the quantity of my cherished emotions like love, joy, and peace? The answer to that question is the same: through Emotional Release Therapy. Through the heart, we can release emotional pain and enhance cherished emotions.

But emotions are not limited to storage in the heart, where they are supposed to remain. Emotions can be stored in all body tissue. From my experience in practicing Emotional Release Therapy, it appears that the cherished emotions of a healthy, happy person are naturally stored in all body tissue. In these persons, destructive emotions are found only in the heart, because destructive emotions are not supposed to be stored anyplace but in the heart.

But if the quantity of destructive emotions becomes too great for the heart to contain, they expand from the heart to the solar plexus and lower abdomen. Then they expand into the organs of the body, such as the liver, lungs, stomach, intestines, pancreas, spleen, kidneys, bladder, sexual organs, and reproductive organs. They can also expand into the muscles, nerves, blood vessels, bones, joints, skin, and soft tissue.

Sometimes the destructive emotions can apparently completely skip the heart, the solar plexus, the lower abdomen, and go directly to a major organ or to one precise area, such as the lower back, neck and shoulders, calf muscles, hands, feet, or joints.

The area where these emotions are stored becomes susceptible to dis-ease or disease. Thus the mind-body connection is not so much the "brain-body" connection, but rather the "heart-body" connection. The heart and the emotions become a major component of all medical conditions.

By removing the destructive elements of this energy, we can restore health to any part of the body. While doing this, we can also enhance the quantity of constructive energy,

We Are Electrical Beings

Every cell in your body is filled with a tiny amount of electrical energy. The brain operates on about one-billionth of a volt. The heart beats on about one-millionth of a volt. We are energy beings. So in this new concept, each cell contains not only DNA biological programming, but also an energy field that contains additional information—emotions as energy.

Research scientists in this field refer to life-giving energy as subtle energy or life energy. All life on earth must be filled with life energy, also known as healing energy, in order to live.

To me, life energy is the divine energy, the creation energy, without which there would be no life on earth. This is composed of (1) the energy that gives life to the DNA biological programming, (2) emotional energy, (3) mental energy, (4) spiritual and moral energy, and (5) the energy of higher consciousness. These energies interact and blend into one cohesive information-bearing, intelligently acting energy—life energy or healing energy.

How did I come up with this new concept? Slowly! I had to work backward from my experiences of removing destructive emotional energy from people and then filling them with constructive life energy, also known as healing energy.

I am not a scientist, but I needed to understand my experiences rationally. So I have created a working model that consistently and predictably explains what is occurring during Emotional Release Therapy. Explaining with consistency and predictability why something works is the basis of all scientific working models.

When I realized that people store their emotional pain in their hearts, not their brains, I developed a means for removing that emotional pain with Emotional Release Therapy (ERT). Then, after an ERT session, a few of my clients complained they still felt the emotional pain in their solar plexus or lower abdomen, and I began to remove emotional pain from those locations with such clients.

People began coming to me with diseased organs, such as the liver, heart, or kidney. After the heart's emotional release, I discovered that diseased organs could release their emotional and physical pain into my hand, bringing health to the organ. With this discovery, I began exploring other possibilities. Anxiety and stress can be released from all the muscles, nerves, blood vessels, and even the skin. When lower-back emotional pain is released, the back pain disappears.

If the feeling of physical pain is released immediately after a physical trauma, the now pain-free trauma-affected cells restore the tissues immediately and the physical trauma disappears before your amazed eyes.

For instance, in South Africa in a game reserve, while it was still dark, I slammed down the tailgate of a pickup truck and caught my fingers between the tailgate and a trailer hitch. It resulted in a terribly painful injury to my fingers. I immediately placed the fingers of my left hand over the injured fingers of my right hand. I asked the right-hand injured fingers to release their pain into my left hand. They did, as I felt the warmth of their release into my left hand. Within 20 seconds, my injured fingers no longer hurt. Using a flashlight, I examined my injured fingers. They had neither bruises nor abrasions. I was shocked. After releasing the physical pain into my left hand, the right-hand fingers had restored themselves to health.

Twenty-five years after I had suffered a heart attack, I asked my heart to release the physical trauma of that moment into my hand, just in case it might still be there. The resulting immense heart-trauma release knocked my hand away from my chest. Wow! My working model was accurate! I immediately asked my plaque-filled coronary arteries to release any physical and emotional trauma. I was shocked by the intensity of the release. It was just as powerful as the previous one from my heart. I then filled both my heart and coronary arteries with God's love and peace, with healing energy. (You will soon learn how do this.)

You can understand why I was fascinated throughout my 11 years of research, discovery, and development. I developed theories to explain what was happening and tested these out on my clients and myself. I concluded that every cell in the body can store emotional and physical pain. How? Emotional pain and physical pain must be carried in information-bearing energy. The pain information in that energy must be at a specific frequency, with each distinct emotional pain having a specific frequency. Each cell must have an energy field in which to store the energy information of each particular emotional and physical pain, as well as the mental, spiritual, moral, and higher consciousness essence of a person.

Emotional Release Therapy is able to help people voluntarily remove destructive information from any cell in the body. Any person can quickly learn to practice ERT and thus be able to help themselves and other people release this destructive storage.

From the beginning, some clients complained that when the emotional pain had been released from their hearts, they felt uncomfortably

7

empty. To respond, I experimented with offering a blessing to fill the void. This was not difficult for me because professionally I am a clergyman who has used ritual and prayer blessings with people for many decades. At first, the blessings were simple. I prayed, "God, fill this person with your love and peace." Afterward, with amazement, I listened to their reports. Each such blessed person reported feeling the qualities of love and peace filling their heart. Some of their faces actually glowed with newfound happiness.

I began experimenting with other qualities in the blessings. I discovered that, with your hand placed on another's sternum or breastbone, you can fill that person's heart with any qualities you can experience or understand, such as courage, boldness, femininity, masculinity, empathy. And that person subsequently feels those qualities within and becomes like those qualities.

I think of John, a single man, who was too shy at 38 to ask a woman at work out on a date. He released his shyness during Emotional Release Therapy. I closed with a blessing like this: "John, be filled with social boldness when talking to this woman." Our time together totaled about 40 minutes. Three months later, John phoned and told me he was engaged to that woman.

Yes, that sounds too simple to be true. Everything I have written so far sounds too simple to be true. But every human value we cherish—love, joy, happiness, and loyalty—sounds too simple to be true.

Comments from readers of my previous books have convinced me that I have the remarkable ability to make the seemingly complex become simple. Like teaching you how to release the trauma of a lifetime of painful memories in an hour or two. Like teaching you to remove destructive emotional states such as depression in an hour or two. Like teaching you to be filled with the emotional qualities you cherish—love, joy, and peace.

Every cell of the body contains energy information about our physical DNA, our emotions, thoughts, spiritual and moral nature, and higher consciousness. In practical terms, this means:

1. Our *physical nature* is not just in our muscles, blood vessels, nervous system, and organs; it is in every cell of the body.

2. Our *thoughts* are not just in our brains; they are in every cell of the body. What we think becomes a part of the information in every cell.

3. Our *emotions* are not just in our hearts; they are in every cell of the body. (But, if intense, emotions can also be stored in specific areas of the body.)

4. Our *spiritual and moral natures* are not only in our brains and hearts, but also in every cell of the body. Their energy emanates from beyond the physical body. For years, I have been able to identify people of high spiritual and moral natures because I can feel the qualities they emanate as absolute peace. As we gaze at each other, we are unified by this peace.

5. Our *higher consciousness,* home of our compassionate dreams and ideals, is not only in our brains and hearts, but in every cell of the body.

So, from the moment of conception, each of these five human traits filters as energy information into every cell of the body. During the various stages of human development (infant, toddler, preschooler, child, youth, adult), all that we are is written into every cell of the human body. This information becomes embedded as intelligently acting knowledge in the total human being.

Why is it important to know this?

Because Emotional Release Therapy must change the way we perceive human development as taking place. What we experience through our family, the classroom, music, TV and movies, religion or spirituality, social interaction, or our community is not just in our brains and hearts. It is in every cell of the body.

This is why our identity—who we are—is so stable. It is written into every cell of the body. This is why it is so difficult for people to grow and change.

Emotional Release Therapy can dramatically change how we transform ourselves and others. Emotional Release Therapy can become the primary tool for human transformation.

Using Emotional Release Therapy, we can remove emotional pain from the heart and all body cells. We can help people voluntarily change their learning potential, thought processes, ingrained beliefs and prejudices, their personalities, and their health.

I had a client who was filled with prejudices and opinions about all

9

kinds of people. It was obvious in just a few minutes of talking to her. After she released her emotional pain with ERT, I spoke to her frankly about her prejudices. I asked, "Would you like to release your prejudices?"

Her reaction astounded me. She answered, "Would I like to release my prejudices? Yes, dear Jesus. They haunt me night and day!" So we did ERT for prejudices. I told her to release a prejudice until she no longer felt it and then go on to another prejudice. It took about 30 minutes. When she was finished, her appearance was completely changed. Peacefulness now emanated from her.

The purpose of religion is to fill the heart and every cell of the body with the essence of God. When this has been accomplished and we are filled with the Spirit of God, our whole being is filled with life-enhancing qualities. Religious rituals transmit a powerful information-filled sacred energy that provides a wall of protection against the dark forces of life. Spiritual journeys may produce similar results. When we take part in religious ritual, worship, or prayer service, the energy of the service permeates our body. We become like the energy of the service. Without consciously thinking about it, this happens, transforming us into the energy generated in the service. This is a transformation just as Emotional Release Therapy transforms. ERT blessings and religious/spiritual rites do the same thing. They fill our cells with life-giving qualities.

It has never before been possible to bless people with specific life-enhancing human qualities. Now we have a means to do this. Now you can easily experiment with how to do this. We can intentionally use our hearts to mold ourselves into the persons we have always wished to become. We can teach others to do the same with Emotional Release Therapy processes. We can enhance religious/spiritual rites to accomplish similar transformation. We can enhance the spiritual journey to do this. But it is not a free trip or cheap grace. It must become a conscious effort and a way of life.

2

Testimonials of Enthusiasm and Joy

This is the testimony of Mary Faktor of Northfield Center, Ohio:

I was in great emotional distress and depression due to breakup of a long-term relationship, when Walter did ERT on me as we spoke on the phone. I felt better, then went to see him that night. I felt much better after our meeting. My depression lifted and I got through the grief of the relationship. I took Walter's seminar and found myself to be a natural healer. I have been performing ERT ever since with great success. I am fascinated by how well it helps people.

I have healed a greatly depressed man whose son had just died. He couldn't function or allow himself to love. His depression immediately ended and his heart was open to love. He has since become engaged and is very happy.

I have worked with a stage-three colon cancer patient who couldn't keep food down after chemotherapy treatments. After one hour of ERT with me, he ate Chinese food for dinner.

I helped a woman going through great depression due to divorce. After ERT, she came out of the depression.

When you practice ERT, you will be blessed. Enthusiasm is wonderful. Even better is spiritual bliss! ERT is often an intensely spiritual experience for both practitioner and client. God is present in this sacred encounter. During ERT, you are also heart to heart with God. This is true for several reasons.

First, emotional pain dulls your awareness of God. When you release your emotional pain, your heart is a more capable receptor of sacred experiences.

Second, as your client releases emotional pain, your heart opens even further in compassion, producing a heightened awareness of holiness and inner well-being. This sacred experience is not fleeting. It may last more than a day.

If you have never experienced God, you will. As Hal of Wadsworth, Ohio, shares:

> ERT is simple and quick, and can be practiced anywhere for immediate and long-lasting results. I do ERT first thing in the morning, just before bed, during sex, while watching TV, while walking, and to achieve peace and calm on airplanes. It is the easiest way for me to achieve peace of mind.
>
> I have used ERT to experience God more fully. I now experience God, and his guidance comes through more clearly. This has led to an overall sense of peace and acceptance of life's problems, whereas before ERT, little things would occupy my mind to the point of extreme discomfort, even suicidal feelings.
>
> Since my very first practice of ERT, I always enter a deep spiritual state while practicing ERT. While at a trade fair in Washington State, my back became very tired. Taking a day off, I drove to the banks of a river, where I dangled my feet in the water while sitting on a picnic table. While practicing ERT on myself, I had a wonderful spiritual and physical healing that has lasted throughout the past two years.

I have led various spiritual and personal growth groups involving, all told, thousands of people. Nothing I ever taught before has been received with more enthusiasm than Emotional Release Therapy. No other subject has caused so many people to practice joyously what I have taught them. Here are the words of some students about their excitement in practicing Emotional Release Therapy.

Carol Adams of Lyndhurst, Ohio, wrote:

> Practicing ERT and physical healing has been the most fascinating and rewarding experience of my life. I'm amazed at how much I enjoy these experiences. And I've found that our efforts to heal others bring wonderful unexpected benefits to ourselves also, like a sense of happiness and peacefulness. People generally notice a feeling of energy when we have completed ERT and state something like, "I feel like I can accomplish anything the rest of this day!"

From Vicki Raymond of London, Ontario, Canada:

> In the first week after Dr. Weston's ERT course, I practiced Emotional Release healing with nine people and also had four sessions with myself. This second week I've had sessions with five people so far. I have had some awesome experiences with this healing.
>
> Let me simply thank you, Walter, for being you! For sharing with us what you know. It is my personal belief that your heart's desires will be manifested in the world—without a doubt—because it is God's will.
>
> This is not so much because of human endeavor, as essential as it is; in spite of us humans, the healing of the world is in process. It's only a matter of time before a more complete healing is attained.
>
> I wish to acknowledge your service and virtues of love, compassion, determination, endurance, and patience with carrying out your life purpose. I thank your wife also for her patience and understanding for your need to travel and share what you know. May God hold you close and guide you always.

(The "Dr." is due to my doctorate in healing research.)

Liz Tekus of Cleveland, Ohio, states:

I was drawn to your Emotional Release Therapy workshop because I was intrigued by the information you presented to our church this morning. I thoroughly enjoyed the seminar and went on to work on three people shortly afterward. Two of these were skeptics—my sister and a teenage boy. I didn't know if either would consent to the process. The third was my husband, who is very receptive to things of this nature. All three released and felt relieved after their sessions.

Marlene of Goderich, Ontario, Canada, e-mailed me a week after the ERT seminar:

Hi, Walt: I have been very busy with setting up my ERT business. I completed my ninth client last night. I am amazed at the results.

My favorite one was a friend that I gave two free sessions to. What I am finding with people on their first session is that they have a lot of intense emotion to release, then on the second session there is not a lot.

What happened in this particular session was that the client released for a while, then I guided her to fill the empty space with love and peace. An overwhelming sense of love and peace came over me also and we were both immersed in it. It was a beautiful feeling that I have rarely felt. It was incredible! Every one of the nine report feeling lighter and peaceful.

Yesterday I had a highly tense and anxious male client. He was very cooperative and released a great deal. He reported feeling peaceful, which is rare for this person. He is a compassionate person to and for everyone but himself. Yesterday afternoon he went out and actually bought himself a ring he has always wanted. Last evening he reported lying down and sleeping for three hours after he got home. This is a person who is in high gear all the time. Amazing!

I also had a 17-year-old boy come for a treatment. I did not sense the intense emotions that I have in more, let's say, mature clients. He released a couple of emotions and he reported feeling peaceful. He is a young man who has a lot going on and felt tired of having so much on his plate.

I am also seeing his mother. Her husband recently left her for another woman. I have seen her twice and she is doing very well. The first time she walked into my office, she looked at the Kleenex box and started crying. She is much more at peace now and even her face has changed. It seems to have softened. This is amazing work.

Oh, and I have a friend in Florida that I practiced doing ERT over the phone with.

What I am experiencing is that two to three sessions take care of the emotional trauma. Pretty inexpensive remedy for years and years of trauma, right?

Thank you so much for sharing your information and gift with me. It has changed my whole life and I can now use the talents I have known I have had for a long time. I wish you all the success and happiness in your life.

Of the almost four hundred people I have used ERT with over the past ten years, I can recall only three people who were not helped. Of my more than three thousand seminar graduates, only a handful could not competently practice ERT after their 12 hours of training. This rate of success brings me ongoing enthusiasm and fulfillment.

When I arrived in Bangalore, India, in 1996, my Hindu pranic healer students expressed concern about their outcomes. Few of their clients were being healed and then only temporarily. The International Pranic Healing Association has trained more than one hundred thousand healers from many faith traditions and nations to practice their energy healing method. To enhance their method, they had invited me to teach them my healing approach. I taught them ERT and touch-healing prayer, although many of them were already using prayer.

After my seminars, my phone barely stopped ringing as they expressed their enthusiasm for Emotional Release Therapy. Using ERT first, they permanently cured almost everyone they practiced pranic healing with. In addition, they were experiencing spiritual joy during their healing encounters.

In September 2000, I had a spirited response in South Africa. Molly and Gordon Bailey, directors of Training and Resources in Early Education (TREE), had invited me. TREE, a nonprofit group, educates 80,000 rural Zulu children, provides community health centers, and develops community gardens.

They had invited me to train Zulu women in the practice of ERT, so these leaders could train the community to remove the trauma of AIDS-orphaned children, who may number in the millions in the coming decade. I trained teachers, supervisors, social workers, and many others.

My biggest challenge with the rural social workers was language. They were literate in the Zulu language, but not in English. So I had to work through a translator, which meant brief instructions. The women were all Catholic and the translator was a Baptist minister.

I need not have worried. They were skillful students who quickly learned and enthusiastically practiced ERT. When I returned ten days later, each social worker proudly beamed as she gave her testimonials of ERT successes.

They had worked with people filled with far more emotional trauma than I had ever seen. Before I left, they began singing in Zulu some of the most beautiful and heart-rending music I had ever heard. Tears of joy glistened on every cheek as they serenaded us out to our pickup truck. I am still moved by this experience as I write this, tears once again flowing joyously down my cheeks. May you move on to the wonder and joy of practicing and experiencing ERT.

Part II

Self-Healing

3

Healing Oneself with ERT

The following story came to me to me in my e-mails: "For 20 years I have suffered with fibromyalgia, allergies, and sinusitis/bronchitis. Three times they have caused me to become ill for most of a year. I knew my conditions were caused by my emotional reactions to life. It was not until I read your book *Healing Yourself* that I found the solution by using Emotional Release Therapy on myself.

"Following the release of my painful memories by using ERT on myself, I was finally able to heal my illnesses and was symptom free within three or four days.

"Thank you, thank you, for sharing your life's work with us. You have given me new life, which I hope to pass on to others. In honor of my 65th birthday, I ordered and sent your books to five of my friends. Jackie."

I have never met or spoken to Jackie, nor do I know where she lives. I replied by sending an e-mail: "Thank You."

As I read this e-mail again, I had the same reaction as I originally had. I was moved by her story of self-healing and tears came to my eyes. My God, she became well for the first time in 20 years! She regained life with ERT. I rejoiced with her. I celebrated with her.

Messages like hers assure me that it is possible for anyone to practice ERT successfully. Hundreds of people have since shared their beneficial experiences. But hers was the first e-mail I received. That was in 1998.

She read about ERT. She tried it. ERT worked for her.

A local massage therapist, asked to write a testimonial for ERT, replied with three words, "It always works!"

It always works. That's what I want to share with you. It always works. Don't be doubtful that such a simple technique could possibly work for you. It simply sounds too wonderful to be true. Have the confidence that it works for everyone, even you. It always works.

Diane Keefe of Valley Park, Missouri, was one of my earliest ERT clients. She later sponsored an ERT seminar. Here is Diane in her own words:

> Self-ERT removes emotional trauma, helpful for safer driving. I went to the grocery store and was running late on beginning a trip. Leaving the parking lot in a hurry, I passed a slow car and entered the left exit lane. The man in the car I had passed came up beside me in the right lane and began yelling obscenities at me, his face distorted with rage.
>
> I cried all the way home. I unloaded my groceries and yelled at my children to get in the car for our trip. I was still upset and realized this was putting my children into danger with my erratic driving. So, as I drove, I practiced ERT on myself. I was immediately calm again and continued on my trip peacefully. A real miracle.

Jeanne Noble of Jeromesville, Ohio, also a former client and student, tells of a similar inner quieting with ERT:

> Recently, my husband and I moved. After three days of packing and unpacking, I realized I was very stressed out. I did ERT on myself to release my anxiety. When I got in touch with the feeling of anxiety, I realized that it was the fear of not doing a good job of moving. It was good old performance anxiety. With that realization, I released the fear using ERT and consciously changed

my attitude. The move was still a lot of work, but now I was in a carefree mood.

One night I had a disturbing dream that I forgot soon after waking, but I remembered the message of the dream. For the first time, I realized that I suffered from performance anxiety. It was such a part of me that I never recognized it in myself before the dream. I present myself to most people as a calm, confident person, which has been my own self-image.

I was able to recall that before many professional tasks I felt anxiety. And the night before an overly busy workday, I often had trouble falling asleep and later slept fitfully.

That morning, I practiced ERT for 20 minutes, releasing various situational performance anxieties. For the next few weeks, anytime I recognized performance anxiety, I spent a few minutes releasing it with ERT. Finally, it was gone. I became more peaceful and energized.

Emotional states often seem to possess us. For me, it was like I had stored a pool of anxiety within me that, under certain circumstances, I would automatically tap into. Through ERT releases, I was able to empty that pool so that there was no anxiety left to draw on.

Many people recognize they have emotional problems and want to be relieved of them. What is the best way to do this? In a seminar where she lived, I provided an effective tool to Jane of London, Ontario, Canada. Here is Jane's account of her experience:

> I decided to try Emotional Release Therapy on myself because of my emotional problems. I needed to release a lot of issues surrounding my childhood, especially sexual abuse and the physical torture endured at the hands of my mother. I needed to let go of all of the pain, as it was impeding my growth.
>
> I found that within a week of learning to practice Self-ERT, I was feeling much stronger. I did it on myself about one to two hours every day. It helped me greatly by releasing the pain of my childhood memories.
>
> I feel much different and much more at peace now. I was having problems with the desire to be dead. Since using ERT, that has greatly diminished. I am overall much happier and more peaceful.

Jane had phoned me about her intentions to practice ERT on herself and I had assured her, "It always works."

Jim of Wadsworth, Ohio, who has had many experiences of ERT, reports:

> I went to Dr. Weston for severe back pain. After back surgery, my spinal pain continued. After one session of ERT, I felt marked improvement and continued to do ERT on myself for greater improvement. My headaches also ended.
>
> ERT improved my life, giving me insight on how to release "baggage" that I had been carrying around for many years, thus healing emotional stress. It allowed my mind to rest and not feel any negative emotions. This gave me mental energy available for healing my back. I believe ERT to be of great value, and it has good results for the simplicity of practicing ERT.

I wrestled with myself about including the following account. It sounds too wonderful and impossible to be true. A part of me wanted to omit it, afraid that the astonishing outcome would turn readers off. Another part of me placed this as the first account of this chapter. My better judgment took over and placed it here. I believe that I must first make ERT plausible before telling this wonderful story of truth and triumph. This should be a lead story on CNN and the headline of every newspaper in the world.

Justin Thomson of London, Ontario, is the living proof that he healed himself of muscular dystrophy. Here is his account in his own words:

> For 12 years, since the age of 12, I had limb girdle muscular dystrophy. I was in constant pain as my muscles deteriorated. I was also severely limited in my body movements. Medical doctors stated there was no cure and death would come to me at about age 30.
>
> I wasn't about to just give up. I took it upon myself to explore health and wellness alternatives. Within this category I found Emotional Release Therapy in *Healing Yourself,* a book by Walter Weston.

I phoned Walter. He didn't know if ERT would cure me, but he promised that it would produce emotional peace.

The pursuit and practice of daily ERT were very enjoyable and the improvements I began noticing were extraordinary. After five months of daily ERT, I was symptom free, totally one hundred percent cured of my muscular dystrophy. A miracle had taken place during the process of Emotional Release Therapy.

This new way of thinking and healing is definitely where our society should be focusing its attention. Now, practicing ERT with others, I have witnessed other people's transformations, as the symptoms of depression, sore muscles, hot flashes, and heart disease disappear. And I have just worked with a few people so far. ERT has changed my life significantly and I will never be the same.

At the beginning, after reading *Healing Yourself*, Justin had phoned and asked me, "Does this really work? Can it cure my muscular dystrophy?"

I answered, "Justin, I don't know. I do know that it will remove your destructive emotions. I do know that there appears to be an emotional component to most diseases." My answer seemed to satisfy him. We then did two ERT sessions over the phone.

Almost a year later, I learned that those sessions were actually the deciding factor in motivating Justin to continue. During the touch-healing prayer part, he said it felt like a bolt of electricity shot through his body, including into his legs, where he had little feeling. It was personal proof that I was offering something pretty powerful. I encouraged him to continue ERT on his own and he did. We kept in regular e-mail contact. I think it is important to have at least one person for encouragement. After three months of ERT, he stated he was about 70 percent cured.

In the process of ERT, Justin changed his whole lifestyle. He gave up alcohol and recreational drugs. He adopted a low-fat diet with plenty of fresh fruits and vegetables. He knew very little about God, but ERT opened his heart, the place where we experience God, so he could have his first awareness of God and begin his spiritual journey. Then he visited a professional healer, a Reiki master, who cautioned him that ERT could not possibly help. He should learn to accept the progress of his disease because it was genetically induced. Justin was so discouraged that he lost most of his physical progress.

Fortunately, Justin e-mailed me about his discouragement. I responded by saying that the healer knew nothing about how healing could make genetic changes. Nor did she know about the crucial role of emotional pain in the progression of disease. Nor did she know that once the emotional pain and physical discomfort are gone, his genetically defective genes could become normal. This is because the healing power of God acts to make all genes healthy. I reminded him of the progress he had made and encouraged him to continue.

Two months later, Justin e-mailed me that he had been symptom free for ten days. He was 24 years old. He told me about the miraculous morning of what he called "Cure Day." He awoke one morning and discovered that for the first time in 12 years he was free of muscular pain. He stood up by himself and felt great. He decided to take his first normal walk.

With his friend Brenda, along with his golden retriever Clifford, he went across the street to a park and they walked. He was overjoyed! Then the soreness began. He had forgotten that he had little muscle mass. He smiled in confidence as he returned home with sore legs, knowing that his date with death at age 30 had been canceled.

That is Justin's account. It is an unbelievable story. It is so unbelievable that most of his loved ones discounted it. They saw that he had been cured of muscular dystrophy. When they first saw him healthy, they said nothing. When he enthusiastically explained how it had happened with ERT, they responded with total disbelief. They could come up with no other explanation, yet it could not possibly be through Emotional Release Therapy.

A number of people with muscular dystrophy have heard Justin's account of self-healing. We have reports of their trying ERT on themselves for a few weeks and then quitting in discouragement. Justin's claim seems too outrageous for the Muscular Dystrophy Association.

A year after his healing, in September 2000, I was invited to South Africa to teach Zulu schoolteachers and social workers ERT, so they could use it with children orphaned by the AIDS epidemic. My sponsors insisted that Justin accompany me. The families of muscular dystrophy patients in

Cape Town invited him to their city. We flew in and conducted a weekend ERT seminar for the muscular dystrophy patients and their families.

After the workshop, we kept in touch with the leaders of the group. Weeks later, we were disappointed by the declining morale. How can you motivate people to practice ERT for an hour or more each and every day, month after month? You must have a deep desire to get well. You must believe that removing emotional pain will alleviate the symptoms of your disease and perhaps cure you. You must believe that ERT will work for you. You must become so excited about your future health that you are motivated to practice ERT daily!

Justin Thomson's father had not believed Justin's original story of healing. But a year later, he was very ill with heart failure. He was desperate and willing to try anything that might help, even ERT. I received the following surprising e-mail from him:

Dear Walter,

We know each other through my son and your student, Justin Thomson.

Back in early April, I was sick—much sicker than I really knew or appreciated. My heart had failed so badly that the doctor was not optimistic about my recovery and was considering putting my name on the transplant-needed list.

My heart was beating irregularly and rapidly, tremendously enlarged, and pumping less than 20 percent of the blood within it to the rest of the body. By early May, I had both pneumonia and a blood clot in my lung.

On April 18, you had e-mailed Justin with advice about healing me. Then Justin traveled to my town and practiced Emotional Release Therapy with me. He showed me how to do it on myself. I have done emotional release almost daily since mid-April.

It is now May 23. I just got off the telephone with my family doctor and he had wonderful news for me. I have made a complete recovery that is "unprecedented," "miraculous," and "one for the medical journals."

I was about to have a heart transplant and today my heart has returned to normal size and is beating regularly and normally.

Over 50 percent of the blood in my heart is now pumped out with each beat.

I am very grateful for your help and hope that I can help others who need healing.

Appreciatively, Jack Thomson, Brighton, Ontario

Jack's report implies that emotional pain within the heart and body tissue is a major factor in the disease process. Removal of the emotional pain permits the body to regenerate healthy tissue. This is the assumption I use when someone comes to me for physical healing.

When I left the hospital after a heart attack in 1975, my cardiologist's prognosis was that the damage to my heart muscle was so extensive that he did not expect me to live through the year. And he could do nothing for me. According to him, there was nothing medical science could do to save my life. This was long before Emotional Release Therapy. But I had an emotional healing another way, through meditative prayer.

At first, I was devastated by this prognosis. Returning home from the hospital, I practiced spiritual disciplines two to three hours each morning. It took two weeks to calm my fear of dying. But I felt no physical relief of my frequent angina. Then, in the sixth week, in the midst of my daily self-healing spiritual disciplines, I had a dramatic healing.

I was lying on my back in bed, doing a healing meditation, when I had a peak experience of God. I felt God's love, joy, peace, and presence completely fill me. A mystical white light filled my mind. Tears of joy flowed freely down my cheeks.

Then something beyond my conscious mind lifted my hands and placed them on my chest. My hands were hot and I could feel them release a healing energy into me that flowed through my whole body. My toes even tingled. I thought, "I wonder if I have been healed." Deep down, I knew I had been, but I was not ready to trust my inner certainty. I had not expected any physical healing from my daily spiritual disciplines. I had been preparing myself for death.

Later, during my three-month checkup with my cardiologist, I recorded a normal healthy EKG (electrocardiogram), meaning my formerly dead heart muscle had been regenerated and was now normal.

My cardiologist was excited. He said, "This is one for the medical books. This has never before been reported in medical journals or at cardiology conferences. You are a miracle patient."

I asked, "Are you going to write this up?"

He replied, "No, no one would believe me."

I responded, "How do you know that this has not happened thousands of times before, but no doctor has dared to report it?"

He was silent.

Today, I know how to restore the damaged heart muscle from a recent heart attack of a client in a just a few minutes.

Reclaiming one's health is a process. For six weeks, I practiced spiritual disciplines for one to three hours daily. The only sign that something good was happening was that, after two weeks, I knew inner peace at all times. I did not expect a physical healing ever to occur. But on reflection, I see now I was setting the stage for my physical healing.

Justin Thomson practiced ERT three hours a day for five months. During that time, there was slow but steady improvement in his muscular dystrophy symptoms. One morning, he awoke to a dramatic relieving of all muscular dystrophy symptoms on his Cure Day, which he celebrated with a walk in the park. Justin was fearful for months afterward that he would have a relapse of muscular dystrophy, so he kept up his daily ERT sessions. The sessions led him on a spiritual journey that forever changed him.

Jack Thomson practiced ERT twice daily for five weeks before his heart was healed. Even though he was trying to heal his heart, he was enormously surprised when it happened.

What I am saying is that with physical healing, a process takes place over a period of time. For Justin, it was five months. For me, it was six weeks. For his father, five weeks. We were each motivated by desperation. No one believed in what we were doing. But we did it. For each of us, our family members were gone for the day so we had time to do what we chose to do, heal ourselves.

Regaining physical health is a process taking place in time. Most emotional pain must be removed with ERT because emotional pain prevents the body from healing itself. It also prevents the healing energy of prayer from doing its miraculous work. So removing emotional pain is a daily process. Healing of a chronic disease condition usually does not occur spontaneously. It is a process taking place in time, a week or a month.

Healing prayer works as a process, needing to be used regularly. Health is restored using ERT and the presence of an ongoing therapeutic level of God's healing power, working to regenerate slowly the health of every cell. The daily discipline of practicing ERT and healing prayer is still needed for a while after all symptoms of disease are gone. The healing process can mask the symptoms of disease so that they are not readily apparent.

(In 2001, I developed a new technique that talks to the cells. It removes both emotional pain and physical dysfunction. I call it ERT BodyTalk. I give instructions for practicing ERT BodyTalk later in this book.)

When local clients come to me, they refuse my suggested daily sessions for three days straight. When I suggest they come back tomorrow, they usually respond, "Let's make it next week." But people who come from out of town and stay in a local motel are far more likely to follow my instructions. If I say we need two sessions a day for four days, they are all willing to do it.

There is a dramatic improvement in symptoms after four to eight sessions. Then I show my clients how to practice ERT when they go home. If they practice ERT, they rarely need to return to me. They have chosen to take responsibility for their own healing. Within one to three weeks, they are symptom free.

After Justin e-mailed me about his cure, I cautioned him to continue his daily ERT work. He was way ahead of me. He continued doing daily ERT for the next 15 months, fearful that if he stopped, his muscular dystrophy might return with a vengeance. When Justin began practicing ERT, he was a pioneer with no directions on what to do to get well. He believes that if he had known then what he now knows, he could have gotten well much more quickly.

Justin Thomson is unique. He is the only person on earth who has practiced Emotional Release Therapy on himself for three hours every day for 20 months. At an average of three hours of ERT a day, that comes out to about 1,800 hours of ERT. The result is that Justin has become extremely empathetic and spiritual.

4

Self-Healing with Basic Emotional Release Therapy

Having emotional pain is like being possessed. Emotional pain has a life of its own beyond our conscious mental control. No matter how we try to shake it off, it clings to us like glue. Most of us learn ways to wall it off from our conscious awareness. This is a necessary normal defense mechanism to protect us from emotional overload.

Some manage emotional pain by closing themselves to all awareness of feelings. This means living only in the thinking mode, so that you have no contact with your emotional self. The heart has become closed to emotions. Some of us are better at this than others. Others fail to suppress successfully and are haunted daily by their emotional pain.

But no matter how well you cope, unresolved emotional pain remains destructive. It can seep through your defenses as nameless anxiety, fear, stress, anger, or depression. Even when you cannot feel them, destructive emotions can make you ill.

Unhealed emotional pain causes diseases that are resistant to both conventional medical care and alternative medical care. As long as your energy fields are distorted by the emotional pain in the emotional energy field, a constant signal is being sent to the physical body to be ill.

If we know we have access to our emotions through the heart, how do we remove them? We can voluntarily release the negative emotions by feeling them and releasing them into a hand on our heart. The hands must be rinsed periodically in saltwater to dissolve the painful emotions, which are toxic. Healers in India have used saltwater for this purpose for centuries during physical healing attempts.

How would you like to release all your emotional pain and destructive emotional states, ending up feeling a sense of inner peace and contentment?

How would you like to wake up each morning happy and joyous about being alive?

How would you like to get well and become completely healthy and whole?

How would you like to be freed from the emotional barriers that have sabotaged your efforts at meeting personal and vocational goals?

These are the amazing promises of Emotional Release Therapy.

Emotional Release Therapy is revolutionary in scope. It will radically alter the way in which healthcare is practiced. Millions of people will now be able to live happy and productive lives after just one or more Emotional Release Therapy sessions. This is only a small part of the Emotional Release Therapy story.

I met an elderly woman while working in a healing center in Bangalore, India. She had expressed no interest in her daughter's healing work, but when her daughter told her about the American who could remove painful memories from throughout a lifetime, she said, "I want to see this Dr. Weston tomorrow!"

The next morning, 82-year-old Mala walked into the healing center. She was stooped over, the weight of a lifetime etched on her lined face. She said not a word. For 40 minutes, she silently released her long history of emotional pain into my hand from her heart. I was amazed by the intensity of her release.

When Mala finished, she arose. I knew her deepest yearnings had been fulfilled for she stood straight and her face looked peaceful and younger. Then she simply stated, "I feel wonderful!" This is the miracle of Emotional Release Therapy.

Here are more examples. After 40 minutes of ERT, a depressed woman felt free, happy, joyous. After ten minutes of ERT, a rape victim was freed of all her emotional and physical trauma. Thirty minutes of ERT erased the emotional trauma of 20 years of being a battered wife.

A combat veteran's life was in chaos due to post-traumatic stress disorder. After two sessions of ERT, he was whole once more, the agony of combat gone.

A woman was in the late stages of breast cancer when she practiced ERT on herself. Six weeks later, an MRI showed she was cancer free.

The yearning runs deep to be at peace, healthy, and whole. Bringing those yearnings into reality is the promise of ERT.

An Overview of Basic ERT

Emotional Release Therapy is very simple. You place your dominant hand flat over your heart. Choose a color and place it in your heart. Release your feelings into the color and thus into your heart. You will feel the emotions entering your hand as heat. That is Basic ERT. Now the details.

Feelings are fleeting, so it is difficult to hold onto any recalled feeling long enough to release it. We overcome this barrier by using a focus. Choosing a color for your focus and placing the color in your heart under your dominant hand is the first step of ERT. The color doesn't matter. Also, you can change colors at any time.

Your emotions are stored in your heart. Releasing *thoughts* of emotional pain cannot release the pain. Thoughts do not produce heat, but only a tingling. You must release *emotions*.

Children can release a lifetime of emotional pain in 15 to 30 minutes. Women generally take 30 to 60 minutes for the release. Thinking-type men tend to take longer.

Before beginning, find a kitchen bowl large enough to place your hand in. Add two tablespoons of salt. Half fill it with hot water. You will be dipping your hand in it for a half-hour or so, so you want the water to remain warm.

The released painful emotions are toxic. When your hand grows very warm, rinse it in the saltwater, which dissolves the toxicity, and then dry your hand with a dish towel. One day, no saltwater was available when I practiced ERT with a depressed woman. That night, I woke up at 4 A.M. very depressed. I got up and sat in the living room for a half-hour doing Emotional Release Therapy on myself until I was at peace. Using saltwater during Emotional Release Therapy with the woman would have dissolved the depression before it entered me.

Everyone has painful memories and troubling emotional states. If you release one troubling emotion, it usually connects you with others for a half-hour or so of release. Even deeply buried ones are released this way. Everyone can do it. Don't let self-doubt stop you.

You may choose to delay the release of some painful emotions. For 16 months, my sister nursed her husband through brain cancer. After his death, I observed her grief, exhaustion, and despair for a month before cautiously offering her Emotional Release Therapy.

She eagerly accepted my offer, as if I should have offered it sooner. Immediately after ERT, she was her old energetic, optimistic self. As a widow, she still had the difficult task of rebuilding her life but was now more capable of doing it.

Practicing Self-Healing with Basic Emotional Release Therapy

1. Begin. Fill a bowl with hot water, pour two tablespoons of salt into the water, and find a towel. Find a quiet place where you will not be disturbed, even by the phone. Lie down so your arm will not grow tired.

2. Ask yourself:

a) Do I have painful memories to release?

b) Do I have an emotional hurt that haunts me every day of my life?

c) Do I daily dwell in any emotional state that makes me unhappy or sabotages my life?

d) Do I daily dwell in any emotional state that makes my loved ones unhappy?

Focus on your answers during Emotional Release Therapy. These answers are the best place to begin.

3. **Your hand.** Begin by placing your dominant hand (right- or left-handedness) flat over your heart. Your hand is capable of receiving the energy your heart releases. Have the bowl of saltwater handy so you can rinse your hand in it when your hand grows warm to dissolve the toxic emotions that will be released into your hand.

4. **Close your eyes** throughout the process, except when reading prayers and directions.

5. **A focus.** Choose the emotion that causes your worst pain. Choose a color as a focus for releasing your chosen emotion. Feel the emotion you are about to release. Visualize your focus and place it in your heart area. Offer a prayer that expresses your intentions.

6. **Prayer.** "God, I no longer want this emotional pain and I choose to release it into my hand. Thank you. Amen."

7. **Release.** Release the focus, the color, into your hand. You might want to view your hand as a magnet or a vacuum, pulling your emotions into it. Or let the color flow like a river into your hand. Or invent your own release mechanism. There may be up to a ten-second delay before you feel the heat of your release entering your hand. Once you learn to do this, try to feel the emotion, letting it flow into your hand with the color. If the color changes, go with the new color.

8. **One emotion at a time.** Release an emotion until you can no longer feel it. It's gone! Then go to another emotion. Release one emotion at a time.

9. **Checking your progress.** If the emotional release is working for you, you will be aware of a heat entering your hand. That is the emotion you are releasing. It is toxic to you.

10. **Rinse your hand in saltwater to dissolve the emotions of your release when your hand feels very warm.** This rinsing is necessary because your hand quickly fills to capacity with released emotional

heat, which is toxic. The rinsing also makes your hand more sensitive, so that you can feel the heat release. Now return your hand to your heart.

11. **A tingling.** If you feel a tingling in your hand, you are releasing thoughts, not feelings. Reach deeper for your emotions.

12. **Nothing.** If you feel nothing entering your hand, start over. This time, try releasing the emotion and/or event directly into your hand. If needed, try releasing the emotion with each exhale.

13. **Still nothing.** If you still feel no energy or heat entering your hand, do not give up. Try to feel something in your hand if it is not heat. You gained some insights in your first attempt. Everyone eventually succeeds.

14. **Finished.** You have finished releasing your emotion from your heart when no further heat enters your hand.

15. **Proceed to other releases.** Keep releasing like this until you have released whatever emotional pain you can find.

16. **Prayer blessing.** Close each session with a sacred blessing. With your hand on your heart, pray: "God, fill me with your love, joy, and peace. Thank you. Amen."

You have completed basic Emotional Release Therapy on yourself.

Help for Insomnia

When you have trouble falling asleep or lie awake in the middle of the night, you can use Emotional Release Therapy to fall back to sleep.

Lie on your back. Place your hand on your heart. Release the emotions of what is keeping you awake, along with stray thoughts (which are feelings). Shake your hand to rid it of toxic emotions.

Then go to your navel with your hand and do the same release there. You are releasing from the solar plexus and lower abdomen at the same time.

Then, with your hand on your heart, pray, "God, fill me with your peace and with sleepiness." Say it three times.

Then, with your hand on your navel, pray, "God, fill me with your peace and with sleepiness." Say it three times.

5

Self-Healing with Advanced
Emotional Release Therapy

Any time you use Advanced ERT, it should be preceded by Basic ERT.
Experiment with these exercises to see what works best for you.

The numbering of steps is a continuation from the last number used
in the previous chapter so that you will not be confused when referring to
exercises by number. So we begin with step 17.

17. **Go to the abdomen.** Move your hand to your abdomen (just below
    your navel) and practice ERT. It is here that gut-level emotions such as
    fear and anger tend to gather. If you feel no release, no emotions are
    stored there. Rinse your hand often in saltwater.

18. **Go to the solar plexus.** When finished with the abdomen, move your
    hand to your solar plexus (just below the ribs) to release any remain-
    ing emotional pain. Rarely will you feel a release, but do it anyway, just
    in case. Rinse your hand often in saltwater.

19. Emotional pain from other people. Family members, friends, and work associates are the most likely source of the worst emotional traumas. With each person, first release anything about the person that irritates you, such as physical appearance, voice, personality, or style. Then release the emotions of any negative feelings you have about these attributes, then any associated with the person, and then any disappointments. Begin with family members, alive or deceased: grandfathers, grandmothers, father, mother, spouse, children, and siblings. Proceed to friends and former friends. Conclude with your work associates and with the responsibilities you find stressful or boring. Remember to rinse your hand in saltwater as needed.

20. Improving your self-image. This an important exercise. Release any feelings about yourself that you don't like, such as your physical appearance, personality, shame, embarrassment, guilt, a sense of inadequacy. Release your feelings about each of these into your hand on your heart. Rinse your hand in saltwater as needed. For example, you might say, "I release my shame about my fat waist." Feel the feeling and release your feelings into your hand. Your purpose is to accept your fat waist rather than finding it repulsive.

21. Hidden emotional pain of gestation and birth. Go to your past. Begin in the womb during your mother's pregnancy. Say, "When I count to one, I will release my emotional pain from when I was in my mother's womb. 3, 2, 1, release." Keep on releasing until there is nothing to release. Rinse your hand. Then go on to a moment of birth trauma. "I release all trauma of my birth. 3, 2, 1, release."

22. Hidden emotional pain from childhood. Begin with kindergarten. Say, "When I count to one, I will release the emotional pain surrounding kindergarten. 3, 2, 1, release." Keep on releasing until there is nothing to release. Rinse your hand. Then go on to each grade: first grade, second grade, third grade, fourth grade, fifth grade, sixth grade. Release the emotional pain of each elementary grade.

23. Hidden emotional pain from youth. Now let's go to your youth. Say,

"When I count to one, I will release the emotional pain surrounding the seventh grade. 3, 2, 1, release." Keep on releasing until there is nothing to release. Rinse your hand. Then go on to each grade—eighth grade, ninth grade, tenth grade, eleventh grade, twelfth grade—and do the same.

24. **Hidden emotional pain in adulthood.** Now let's go to adulthood. Say, "When I count to one, I will release the emotional pain surrounding the ages 18 to 25. 3, 2, 1, release." Keep on releasing until there is nothing to release. Rinse your hand. Then go on to each five years, ages 25–30, 30–35, and so on.

25. **Emotional pain you remember from the past.** Go back through every painful time in your life and release the emotional trauma of it. Recall moments of rejection, blame, shame, embarrassment, grief, failure, broken relationships. If you cannot feel the emotions of the moment, try to relive it and imagine what your emotions would have been. Begin with childhood. If there is a hurt you recall every year or two, go to it. You recall it because it is emotional pain. Pray, "I release my hurt into my hand. Amen."

26. **Cutting emotional ties.** If you have people in your past or present who haunt you with painful emotions, you probably have a cord of energy binding you to them. This energy bond may be with a parent, grandparent, an estranged or deceased spouse or lover, a spouse, a child, a sibling, a friend, a coworker, or whomever. Cutting your energy ties to them can stop your emotional discomfort and give you a new sense of freedom. Do this exercise one person at a time. Visualize a cord of energy connecting you to him or her. Then take an imaginary pair of scissors and cut this connecting cord to sever any energy contact with that person. While doing so, pray, "God, I cut this cord that binds me to _____. May the bond between us be completely severed that I might be at peace with him/her. Thank you. Amen."

27. **Past lives.** Past lives is a term referring to previous lives that your soul has experienced in other physical identities of which you have no

memory. Some people believe that the trauma and sin (karmic debt) in one's past lives harmfully influence one's present life. Whether or not you believe in past lives, I urge you to experience the possible positive effects of this exercise on you. With your hand on your heart, tell yourself, "When I count to one, I will release into my hand all the karmic debt of my past lives that is harming my present health and development. 3, 2, 1, release." If you feel a strong release, repeat this exercise. Rinse your hand as needed.

Conclusion

These are your advanced options for practicing Emotional Release Therapy on yourself. You may develop others. If you are just seeking the release of your emotional pain, the exercises in this and the previous chapter are all you need. How long you'll need in order to release all your emotional pain is unknown. An hour, three hours, six hours. If it is childhood trauma, it takes longer.

If you remain in an unhappy relationship at home or at work, you may need to practice ERT often. You may be able to improve your relationships by practicing ERT with loved ones and work associates. This may remove all the negativity between you. If it does not, suspect that you or the other person is holding onto feelings such as anger, fear, distrust, and resentment. You may need to separate yourself from persons who continually raise negative emotions in you.

I once practiced ERT with a woman who had late-stage breast cancer. But her husband's nastiness was causing her emotional pain. I told her if she were to save her life, she must leave her husband, but she refused to do this because she loved him.

About six weeks after several Emotional Release Therapy sessions had led her to inner peace, she had an MRI that showed she was free of cancer. We celebrated her cure.

Then her husband became the nastiest he had ever been. The cancer returned with a vengeance. During her last week of life in the hospital, she finally expressed all her anger with her husband. But it came too late and she died.

6

ERT BodyTalk for Physical Self-Healing

For permanent results, these physical self-healing exercises must be practiced only after using Basic and Advanced ERT as described in the previous two chapters.

Most conditions respond well to ERT BodyTalk. After daily practice, within a week or two, all symptoms are gone. Doing this requires a desire to get well, trust in the process, and discipline. If you wish to regain your health, these exercises must become a daily priority. Regaining your health enhances the pleasure and attainment in every one of your other priorities. If you should falter or dislike practicing self-healing, try using ERT to remove the emotional blockages that cause this. You are worth every minute you use to get well.

Like learning any new skill, ongoing experience provides confidence. Touch-healing prayer will work for everyone who follows the processes. With practice, it becomes as easy as washing dishes. Relax! God's in charge! God works through anyone who follows the described processes.

I again remind you that the following instructions must be preceded by Basic and Advanced Emotional Release Therapy. ERT places all the body cells at peace, allowing the healing energy frequency to be fully received so that it can easily regenerate healthy tissue.

Practicing ERT BodyTalk for Physical Healing

Using BodyTalk with One Diseased Body Part

You can do this specifically with any diseased place in your body. For instance, if you have a diseased liver, talk to your liver with your hand on your heart. Say, "Liver, release your emotional pain, your physical pain, and your dysfunction into my heart and then into my hand. Also release the pain from areas surrounding you, liver." When the heat stops entering your hand, rinse your hand in saltwater. If the release is strong, repeat this procedure.

Then place your hand on top of your head. Say something like this: "God, send your healing power into my brain. Brain, open a door and let the healing power in. Let it flow through you, brain, healing all your functions.

"Now let the healing power flow down through my neck and right lung into my liver. Heal my liver. Restore every cell in my liver to normal and make my liver healthy and whole. Heal the surrounding tissue of the liver. Recreate and make all tissue new and normal. Thank you for the healing that is taking place."

Leave your hand on top of your head for ten minutes. Do this every day for seven days. You may be healed on the first or second day, but you are taking precautions and doing it for seven days.

With this process, you fill your whole body with God's healing power.

Cell Cleansing

Hand position: We are going to cleanse every cell in your body. Close your eyes. Place your dominant hand on your heart.

Talk to the body one organ at a time: Say, "Brain, release your emotional pain, your physical discomfort, and your dysfunction into my hand when I count to one. 3, 2, 1, release."

The release is delayed compared with ERT. If the release is strong, repeat the procedure.

Do this with the brain, ears, eyes, sinuses, nose, throat, lungs, heart, liver, pancreas, spleen, esophagus, stomach, intestines, bladder, kidneys, reproductive organs, sexual organs, nerves, muscles, bone joints, blood vessels, blood, skin, and so on. Rinse your hand in saltwater.

Say, "Release your emotional pain, your physical discomfort, and your dysfunction into my hand when I count to one. 3, 2, 1, release."

Filling Your Body with God's Healing Power

Hand position: Close your eyes. Place your dominant hand on top of your head. Your hand will become less tired if you are lying down.

Pray: "God, may your healing power flow from my hand into my brain. Thank you. Amen."

Talk to the brain: Say, "Brain, open a door and let this healing flow in." Mentally visualize it flowing into you.

Talk to God: "God's healing power, flow throughout my brain, restoring all brain functions and filling them with your peace. Amen." Imagine it flowing throughout your brain.

Do the same with the other body organs: Eyes, ears, sinuses, nose, mouth, throat, lungs, heart, liver, gallbladder, pancreas, spleen, esophagus, stomach, intestines, bladder, kidneys, reproductive organs, sexual organs, nerves, muscles, bone joints, blood vessels, blood, skin, and so on.

With your dominant hand on the top of your head, pray, "God, may your healing power flow from my hand into my _____. God's healing power, flow throughout my ____, restoring my health and filling it with your peace. Amen."

Imagine it flowing throughout your _____ [body part].

Healing Body Sections

Place your hand on top of your head and pray, "God, may your healing power flow from my hand into my brain, renewing every cell in my head, flow down my right arm into my fingers, renewing every cell in my right arm, flow down my left arm into my fingers, renewing every cell in my left arm, flow from my brain down my throat into the whole torso, renewing every cell in my torso, flow down my right leg to my toes, renewing every cell in my right leg, flow down my left leg to my toes, renewing every cell in my left leg. Amen."

Charged Healing Towel

For selective body healing, charge a cotton dish towel with the healing energy. Fold the towel into a small shape and hold it between your hands. Pray, "God, fill this towel with your healing power that it might provide me with healing. Thank you. Amen."

Charge the towel in your hands for about ten minutes. While charging it, you can talk, watch TV, or read, because your hands know what to do. Fold the towel to the desired size. Place it on the bare skin in the area needing healing. Secure with your clothing or, if the area is on a limb, use rubber bands loosely around the towel to hold it in place. Let it remain there 24 hours a day. It is releasing healing energy, like an IV sends healing medicine and nutrients into your body.

You will know it is filling you with the healing flow by the slight heat you will feel under the towel. The towel loses its healing energy as it heals. Recharge it once a week.

I have successfully used this with trauma injuries, arthritis, angina, diseased organs, skin diseases, surgical wounds, sore throats, sinus infections, and sunburn.

Charged Healing Water

You can fill water with healing energy, just like you did a towel. With both your hands, hold a gallon jug or other container of water. Pray, "God, fill this water with your healing power so that the water will heal my body. Thank you. Amen." Hold it for 15 minutes. While holding it, you can talk, watch TV, or read. Your hands know what to do and need no further effort on your part. After you have charged the water in this way, drink two ounces of it at a time with every meal and at bedtime. The water will release healing energy into every cell. Continue drinking the water until three days after all symptoms are gone.

I used this with Gertrude, an 86-year-old woman who had spurs (calcium deposits) on her spinal cord. She had been an invalid, unable to walk because of the pain. After drinking healing charged water for four days, she was symptom free until her death at 93.

Localized Conditions

If the condition is due to an injury, surgery, or a disease present in one location in the body, use the following process. The sooner you practice healing with a trauma injury, the more quickly symptoms disappear. An immediately treated sprained ankle will have no symptoms within five minutes. Deep auto accident bruises on the thigh can be gone in a day.

1. **Remove the trauma.** Place your dominant hand about one-quarter inch above the skin. Talk to that location, saying something like, "Release your emotional pain, your physical discomfort, and your confusion into my hand." You may or may not feel the heat of the release. Hold your hand there for about a minute. Then either shake your hand to rid yourself of the body's release or dip it in a bowl of saltwater.

2. **Practice healing.** Place your hand on the skin. If the location is on an arm or a leg, use both hands, one on either side. Offer a prayer, like "God, may your healing power flow through my hand and into my body. Make every cell become normal and fill them with your peace. Thank you. Amen." Hold your hand(s) there for about a minute.

3. **Open your body.** After the prayer, talk to your body. Say, "Open a door under my hand and let the healing flow in." Sometimes you will feel your body's immediate intake of the healing energy. This can feel like a whoosh, as the body sucks it in.

4. **Assess.** Remove your hand and then shake it. Then return your hand to the area. If your hand remains cool, the tissue has been filled with all the healing flow it needs and you are finished with this session. If the hand grows warm, more healing energy is needed; keep your hand there for another two minutes. Check your progress again by shaking your hand and replacing it to assess the need. You are now finished with this phase of healing.

5. **Repeat.** Do this process twice a day until all the symptoms are gone.

These are all the ways in which physical healing takes place.

Part III

Healing Others

7

Testimonials about Physical Healing in Practicing ERT with Others

Here are accounts of practicing ERT for the physical healing of others. You, too, can do physical healing.

Here's Jim Beasley of Atlanta, Georgia, in his own words:

I have been practicing ERT and healing touch with clients and family for almost two years now and have had wonderful results.

I had a friend of mine visiting from California last year. We decided we would go for a walk at a local national park in the Atlanta area. We had been walking for almost an hour and we were a long way from any help when my friend was stung by a wasp or a hornet. Thank God he wasn't allergic to the venom, but almost immediately his finger began to swell.

We walked a few yards more when the thought occurred to me to use ERT on the sting. By this time, the hand was beginning to swell and my friend was in a lot of pain. I asked him if I could do

ERT on his fingers and hand. He was skeptical but agreed. Within a few minutes, the pain began to decrease and the swelling reduced. Within ten minutes, the pain and swelling were almost gone.

As we walked back to the ranger headquarters, the swelling was limited to the tip of the finger where the wasp had stung him, and the pain was nominal. He said he'd always wanted to experience a miracle of healing and he did that day.

Jim also shares this story about his daughter's healing: "My daughter was visiting Atlanta from North Carolina and had just had her second child. She woke up one morning and was complaining of a pain in her breast. My wife, who is an RN, examined her and said it was a stopped-up milk gland. I asked my daughter if I could do ERT on her. She agreed. Within a very short period of time, the pain stopped and the gland reopened."

Dr. Calvin Hawn of London, Ontario, Canada, states:

You may be interested in my experience with ERT in my dental practice. Since taking your workshop, I have included ERT as part of my routine practice after invasive procedures, such as extractions, fillings, and various other surgeries.

On completion of the procedure, I take a minute to ask the patient to close her/his eyes and, without comment or explanation, place my hand or fingers near the affected site. I then visualize the tissue and talk (silently) to it, asking it to release any trauma it has suffered into my hand. When I have a sense that the release is complete, I then direct healing energy into the tissue, asking that it be restored to health and experience no pain. Walter, I can honestly state that the amount of postoperative pain experienced by my patients has dramatically reduced.

Ken McDonald of Wooster, Ohio, didn't tell me of his medical problems until I asked for reports for this book. Here is his story:

When I went to my first ERT session with Dr. Weston, I had gluten intolerance, gout, carpal tunnel, and arthritis. ERT removed my anxiety, definitely cleared my emotions, alleviated my physical symptoms, and gave me an alternative therapy that saved my hands, so I can use them professionally as a massage therapist. And the salt bath was incredible. I felt like a foot of fat just fell off me and into the tub. I did a good ERT release.

Margaret Saraceno of Southbury, Connecticut, tells of her journey back to health:

> Fourteen years ago I came down with fibromyalgia, which filled me with constant severe pain throughout my body plus immense fatigue. I was filled with hope after reading one of Dr. Weston's books. I contacted him and flew to Ohio for Emotional Release Therapy. It was probably one of the best investments and treatments I have ever experienced. Afterward, my physical pain dropped by at least 90 percent. It did not cure my fibromyalgia, but with my own daily use of ERT, it is almost unnoticeable, so I can live as normal a life as possible. I am now using Emotional Release Therapy on others with great success.

Linda Schiller-Hanna of Medina, Ohio, tells how ERT helped her stop pulling her hair out:

> I sought ERT from Walter Weston because I knew someone who raved about his healing work and I also was impressed with his book. I told Walter my biggest problem was something that I had had for over 30 years. I had gone to many different therapists and tried countless remedies with no success.
>
> The problem is called trichotillomania. It is the compulsion to pull one's hair out by the roots, often resulting in bald patches. It had been the source of deep shame and sadness for years.
>
> The day he worked on me, I lay on my massage table and Walter sat beside me with his hand on my heart area and began to lead me through the ERT process. I was amazed. It was a completely new idea to me and it was working. At a certain point, something happened that I will never forget. Suddenly, it was

almost like a bolt of lightning struck me . . . as if a kind of "evil spirit" flew out of my body and across the room and hit the wall. I immediately began to sob with relief. It's as close a thing to an exorcism as I have ever seen on myself or anyone else.

As I am a holistic healthcare practitioner and widely read and experienced in this field, I don't doubt that something highly significant happened. Following this very deep cathartic process, I felt lighter and freer than I had in years. I sensed in Walter a profound caring and faith that is rare in this world. Whether it was his personal abilities or the process or just an excellent tool in the hands of a healing master, I don't know for sure . . . but it worked beautifully.

I was so grateful, I gave Walter my prize possession. It was an eagle feather that had been given to me by a client from Alaska who had had it dropped at his feet when he walked a barren island as the eagle flew over . . . and he had kept it for years himself. To turn over something I treasured that greatly shows the enormity of this experience. I have never regretted the decision to pass on that special item.

For several days after, I did not pull my hair at all. I also suffer from ADD [attention deficit disorder], and for my entire life, I have had an unfinished pile of ironing to do. The day after Walter's work with me, I was able to focus and do all the ironing in the house. It is not that the ironing work is hard for me, but that I would get too restless to complete it . . . or any other project for that matter.

The healing was not entirely complete . . . I have had some residual flare-ups with the hair-pulling, but it has dramatically decreased. I was so impressed with Walter's system that I hosted one of his seminars in my home. There, everyone seemed to learn ERT easily.

When Pat of Columbus, Ohio, came to me, she told me she was suffering daily from severe asthma attacks. Here is her account: "My mother learned about ERT at a service conducted at the Summit Spiritual Center. Dr. Weston was the speaker. My health had been improving over the past two years, but I still required daily medication for my asthma. After ERT I didn't need any medication for about a week. I didn't have to use my inhalers as much as before. I am looking forward to my next session with Dr. Weston." I haven't seen Pat again.

Dr. Hawn used several of the skills I taught him to produce the following account: "A 70-year-old man I was visiting was experiencing neck pain to the point of setting up an appointment to see his physician. I did ERT locally on his neck only, followed by hands-on healing. I then charged a towel with healing energy and advised him to wear it for a couple of days, including sleeping with it. I received a call two days later to tell me he was much improved and had canceled his doctor's appointment."

Placing These Testimonials in Perspective

I am thankful to my students and clients for sharing such a variety of ERT experiences with you. Ninety percent of my own clients need only one or two sessions of ERT to release all their emotional pain and to regain their health.

People who are in the late stages of their diseases usually require ongoing sessions, as do people who have had a chronic condition for a long time. Unfortunately, most people do not seek alternative healthcare until all medical treatment has proven unsatisfactory.

If, immediately after the diagnosis, a woman seeks a cure for her benign or cancerous breast tumor, using the skills you learned in this book, the tumors may disappear. The same is true after early treatment of most medical conditions, including trauma injuries.

I once received a call from a local woman who had just been diagnosed with breast cancer. She could not understand how ERT could benefit her, so I mailed her one of my books. Three weeks later, she phoned me. Jan said:

> I got to the place in your book where it said that about 18 months before the onset of cancer, many cancer patients suffer an emotional trauma. I immediately knew how to cure myself. Eighteen months ago, my only child, a high-school senior, had left home after a terrible argument. I phoned him in Florida and said, "John, this is your mother. I love you. Let's make up." We did.

> The following week I had the cancer surgery on my breast. To his amazement, the surgeon discovered no cancer, only healthy tissue. Thank you, Dr. Weston.

I receive many late-stage cancer patients, whose only other option had been death. They come to me with cancers of the brain, lungs, liver, intestines, bladder, uterus, spine, and others, which have usually spread beyond their initial locations. A few have died, but most of these people are cancer free today, thanks to ERT and ERT BodyTalk.

The testimonials you have read are about quick and dramatic returns to health. With more advanced medical conditions, my basic tool is Emotional Release Therapy, followed up by ERT BodyTalk, used on a continuing basis until health is achieved.

People who come to me from out of state respond the best. They stay in a motel and we are able to do two-a-day sessions for two, three, or four days. Many of them are cured by the time they leave. As with all clients, I teach them how to use ERT on themselves, as well as healing prayer, and urge them to practice these daily. When possible, I also teach family members these skills to use with the client.

8

Testimonials about Emotional Healing in Practicing ERT with Others

These testimonials are from my seminar graduates who tell of their experiences of practicing Emotional Release Therapy to heal emotional wounds. I share these stories to encourage you to practice ERT with others. The emotional healings are exciting.

Claire came to me as a battered wife. For 23 years, she had been emotionally and physically battered by her husband, who had a pool of rage within him. She finally left him, going to a battered women's shelter two years before she came to me, getting a job, and trying to rebuild her life. But she couldn't rebuild her life because she was haunted daily by her past emotional pain from her ex-husband.

As Claire sat down, I wondered if ERT could reach the depths of her despair. She began releasing into my hand hot emotional pain. I've never had anyone who was so ready and capable of release. She released strongly for 40 minutes and then was finished.

She was exhausted by her release, yet her face was peaceful and happy. Claire remarked, "I haven't felt so good since I was a child." Claire contacted me a month later and said, "I still feel wonderful and my life is coming together fast."

Carol Adams of Lyndhurst, Ohio, helped a crime victim. Her account:

A friend of mine was robbed at gunpoint one Sunday morning in the parking lot of a local department store. The next day at work she told me she was very angry about the incident that had ruined her Sunday. She hadn't slept well that night and by Monday morning was having difficulty getting her work done.

I met with my friend at the end of that workday. By that time, she was no longer angry but was feeling tired and depressed. Her eyes were red from crying. After only ten minutes of Emotional Release Therapy, my friend's entire mood changed. As she stood to leave, she said, "I feel good, really good! I feel so light!" Her anger and depression were completely gone. She commented that she knew she could go home, play with her daughter, and enjoy her evening. Several months later, she still reported no emotional trauma, anger, or depression from that incident.

Linda of Canton, Ohio, sent me this e-mail: "Hi, Walter. Thanks for last night's ERT session. My depression is gone and my aches and pains are much better. I feel better, lighter today than I have for a long time."

The next week I practiced ERT with Linda's two teenaged sons. Like many other former ERT clients, Linda attended my next seminar. She now practices ERT with others and meets regularly with a group of ERT practitioners in her community.

One spring morning, I had breakfast with Frank, a Baptist minister from Cleveland, Ohio. I enjoy talking with appreciative readers of my books and with clerical colleagues. Frank was both. Like old friends, we talked about the practice and merits of ERT.

But Frank had some needs of his own and, as we were leaving the restaurant, he made an appointment for Emotional Release Therapy. After our ERT sessions, Frank sent me the following e-mail. "You did ERT twice with me while I was on Prozac for depression. I felt much better after both sessions and am now functioning normally. I soon will be announcing my divorce to my congregation."

Then Frank told about helping a little boy. "I have practiced ERT on a six-year-old boy. His mother brought him to me because he would cry every time she'd get in the car and go away, afraid that she'd get into a car accident and never come back. This was three weeks ago and he no longer cries like this."

Frank learned to practice ERT in two ways. He followed the detailed directions in one of my books as well as experiencing Emotional Release Therapy as a client.

Dr. B. W. of Los Angeles, California, sent me his experience with ERT: "I had been deeply depressed and down on life, mostly because of the death of my father, when Walter Weston practiced Emotional Release Therapy with me over the phone from 2,500 miles away. After we worked together for about 45 minutes, ERT did help by clearing out a lot of depression and gave me a new lease on life."

A seminar graduate, Sharan Robinson of Pennsylvania, sent me this ERT account:

> As a registered nurse, I initially used Emotional Release Therapy in nutritional counseling. One day it went far beyond nutritional counseling. A young woman came to me suffering from severe depression and headaches. She was a new teaching graduate and her depression was so debilitating she was unable to apply for a job as a schoolteacher.
>
> After several ERT sessions, her depression was gone, as were nine years of constant headaches. She also had a noticeably brighter affect. She is now working a full-time job and only has headaches occasionally.

Whatever a person voluntarily releases is gone from them. It usually takes one session, but it can occasionally take several. The primary goal of most Emotional Release Therapy clients is to release their emotional pain. For many, the subsequent release of physical symptoms is a wonderful bonus.

Mary Faktor of Northfield Center, Ohio, gives this account. "I have healed a greatly depressed man whose son had died. He couldn't function or allow himself to love. He has since become engaged and is very happy and no longer depressed. I have worked with a stage-three colon cancer patient who couldn't keep food down after chemo treatments. After one hour of ERT with me, he ate Chinese food for dinner."

Another of my students, Jan Myers of Coshocton, Ohio, sent me a testimonial about her dying father-in-law.

> My father-in-law, Charlie, cut himself off from family members many years ago. My husband, Alan, and I were with him as he was dying. I think only the fear of dying kept him alive. His eyes had been glazed over for several hours when I practiced ERT with him.
>
> In a semi-coma, he released his pain, fear, and anger into my hand. He soon became much more peaceful and his breathing was easier. We told Charlie we loved him and he responded by whispering, "I love you." This was the first time my father-in-law had ever said this to his son, Alan. Then he was gone.

Jan continued:

> Mindy, a young mother with a baby, came to me because of anxiety. Her problems were affecting her emotionally. She was so anxious that she hadn't been able to eat or sleep for several weeks. Mindy agreed to ERT. I couldn't believe how much emotional pain she released with heat into my hand. Afterward, she said, "I can't believe how much better I feel." She then fell asleep for a while. Awaking, she was like a different person. She was talking calmly and ate dinner. The next day she reported that she had slept all night.

Dr. Calvin Hawn of London, Ontario, shared his first experience of practicing ERT: "A 24-year-old female friend of mine is currently experiencing overwhelming emotional distress. I did one session of ERT and she reported feeling relief for two days before feeling overwhelmed again. I gave her your book to read and performed another ERT session yesterday. When we finished, she told me that she felt very centered and grounded."

Faith Strand of Medina, Ohio, tells of her suffering and recovery:

When I met Walter Weston, I was suffering from depression, extremely high anxiety, panic attacks, agoraphobia, fear, phobias, chronic fatigue syndrome, and living in extreme pain and unhappiness in my marriage.

I did not have the energy to visit my parents and friends or to do simple household work like loading the dishwasher. I was a prisoner in my own home, spending my life lying down and sleeping 14 hours a day.

Following many sessions of Emotional Release Therapy with Walter, ERT has taken away the depression and the feeling of emotional overload that I have felt for years.

My emotional pain and anxiety are gone. Since childhood, my phobias with snakes, elevators, and storms have terrified me, but now they are completely gone. Twelve years of panic attacks have disappeared. My physical body has responded to the release of my emotional pain through increased stamina. My blood sugar is now normal.

It is incredible how ERT works! The emotional pain that had been stored inside me since childhood was released! I feel like a huge weight has been taken off my shoulders and I can now feel happiness and joy. It is so wonderful to live in peace. I am thankful every day for Emotional Release Therapy! ERT has enabled me to make enormous decisions about my life that I am sure will change my life forever!

Seminar graduate Melissa, a naturopath from Pittsburgh, Pennsylvania, reports her work with an overwhelmed teacher: "I practiced ERT with a troubled second-grade teacher. The teacher was very frustrated with her class, especially with one student's behavior, and angry about the attitude of his parents. During Emotional Release Therapy, she released her anger and frustration about the situation. Afterward, she reported that she now had better control in her classroom. In a conference with the parents, they worked out a plan to improve the student's behavior and study habits."

Here, Linda Schiller-Hanna of Medina, Ohio, tells us about a touching encounter:

A friend I was visiting in a nursing home mentioned that a fellow resident was in deep grief over her roommate's death the night before. I found this poor woman sitting forlornly in her doorway in a wheelchair. I shared my sympathy with the lady and held her hand. I put my hand on her heart and led her through ERT.

I immediately felt the warmth of her released grief entering my hand. She began crying softly and I could see her face soften and relax as time went by. We only had a few minutes, but I worked as quickly and effectively as I could. When we finished, her face was radiant. She gave me a beautiful smile and she stated, "Thank you. I am at peace." That is the miracle of Emotional Release Therapy.

Allison of Akron, Ohio, read one of my books, then made an appointment for ERT with me. I asked her if she knew what she needed to release and she said yes. We immediately began practicing Emotional Release Therapy. I had no idea what she had come to see me about until she gave this account:

I was suffering from grief, anxiety, and the pain from a relationship when Dr. Weston practiced ERT with me. During our session, I felt a release of a negative, heavy energy. The results continued over time. Now I feel healed of the issues that led me to seek ERT. I was drawn to ERT because I believed in Dr. Weston's credibility. I knew that, with his help, I could learn to take care of my health in a meaningful way through ongoing release of emotional residue and also utilize the practice of ERT to prevent the buildup of emotional debris that blocks healthy energy flow.

During ERT with Dr. Weston, I was able to release longstanding resentment in two close relationships, restore normal elimination, be freed of daily anxiety and intermittent depression. Now, two months after my only ERT session, I consider myself healthy and empowered to continue releasing and healing issues that arise in my normal daily living. I feel a confidence and strength that had been dormant for some time. I am thankful for the emotional release experience and for Dr. Weston's commitment to his work.

I do not need to know the details about the emotional pain of my clients. Many people have difficulty sharing their problems with others. But she sent me her account when I requested accounts for this book.

Emotional Release Therapy is about trusting that people will know what pains them. It is about maintaining privacy and dignity. ERT is about empowering people to feel good about resolving their own emotional pain. It is about being freed to be joyfully happy. Emotional Release Therapy is about confidence in moving into the future.

Ken Kline of Akron, Ohio, shares this account:

> I had suffered with anxiety and panic attacks since childhood. After several sessions of ERT, my anxiety is almost nonexistent. I also use ERT for soul-searching on my spiritual journey. It makes me want to strive to be closer to God.
>
> Walter, you have become a big part of my life, helping me with my spiritual growth and letting the free love of God flow. The line I would use for you is "a priest with the gift of healing."

Today, Karen, 54, came to me to deal with the enormous loneliness she had been feeling in the five years since her divorce as well as the emotional pain from the 24 years of dysfunctional marriage. She released these emotions for about 40 minutes and felt lighter afterward.

I then inquired about her childhood. Karen replied she had no memory of her childhood. To me, this implied that her childhood had been so painful that she had blocked off these memories. So using advanced ERT techniques, we went back to her childhood. During 15 minutes, she had huge releases of emotional pain from preschool and childhood years, as well as lesser releases from her youth.

I knew nothing of what specific emotions she released nor anything about the events that had wounded her. That is the beauty of ERT. It does not matter what occurred in childhood. The details no longer matter because most of the pain is now gone. All the ghosts of the past have been released. In comparison to the current psychological processes of trying to figure it out, this is a far simpler and less agonizing approach with permanent results.

Diane, a woman in her forties, looking tense and forlorn, came to me because she had a troubled marriage. During ERT, Diane released all her emotional pain. I then led her into releasing her negative emotions regarding her husband. These included anger, fear, frustration, and disappointment. Afterward, Diane said, "I wanted my husband, Duane, to come, but he wouldn't."

So I responded, "Tell your husband that there is no need for him to tell me anything about him or your marriage." That evening, Duane phoned for his appointment.

When he came to me for ERT, he said no more than ten words during our hour together, indicating that he was a private, introverted person. He released his negative feelings toward his wife and then I guided him into releasing any negative feelings he had toward himself, giving him, perhaps for the first time in his life, a good self-image. Afterward, he gave me a timid smile, quietly said thanks, and left.

A few months later, I had a chance encounter with Diane at the supermarket. She seemed to be glowing with happiness. She gushed, "Thank you so much, Dr. Weston. My husband is so changed that it is unbelievable. His anger and meanness are gone. For the first time in our marriage, he actually talks to me. We have never been happier. And he liked you."

I had specialized in marriage and family counseling as a pastor, and about 90 percent of the time, it was only with the wife, as most husbands refuse counseling. With no self-disclosure being necessary, I now work with a lot more husbands using ERT.

Beth Donahue of Lakewood, Ohio, shared her account of using ERT for sexual abuse. "I practiced ERT with a woman who had been sexually and physically abused by her father for years. She was able to release her trauma and years of sadness in one session. I closed with a love blessing. Afterward, the woman stated, 'I can now feel responsible for myself. I finally know what love feels like inside!' She looked and acted different after that session."

This is the story of Michelle Gippin, Akron, Ohio:

I sought Emotional Release Therapy about a year after my boyfriend committed suicide. I was experiencing depression, grief, chronic fatigue, repeated respiratory infections, and back problems. I knew they were emotionally based because I had always been healthy before the suicide.

When I met with Walter Weston, we talked about my problem. He helped me get ready to let go of the guilt I was carrying and forgive myself. He practiced Emotional Release Therapy with me for about an hour. As I released my emotional pain, I felt a lot of heat being released from my heart area.

The next day, I was symptom free and have been ever since. I had tried many other treatments, none of which brought me any relief. I am deeply grateful to Walter Weston and Emotional Release Therapy.

Two months later, Michelle phoned me with an update. She was delightfully happy and said that for the first time in her life everything she planned succeeded. Her personal life was coming together. Vocationally, she was achieving beyond her wildest dreams. Five years later, I saw Michelle again while preaching at her church. She seemed to glow with vitality and happiness.

No other approach offers years of extended happiness after an hour-long session. Not psychotherapy! Not medications! Just one session of Emotional Release Therapy can abolish years of depression.

Dana of Norfolk, Virginia, tells this heartwarming story:

After taking your Emotional Release Therapy seminar and experiencing the healing effects, I have lost over 80 pounds this year and my heart's goals are becoming clearer every day. My health has improved and my energy is in abundance. My diet is no longer considered a diet but a way of life.

People who know me have seen a dramatic change in me and my way of thinking. I am considering a move to California and separating from my husband of 16 years. This is a big step for me, but for the first time in my life I am listening to my heart. Many around me disagree with my decision and are trying to hold me back. I will be of greater value to others if I feel free to live and to love.

9

Preparing to Practice ERT with Others

Practicing Basic ERT on others is a simple technique that anyone can accomplish with competence after just a few hours. In my 12-hour ERT seminar, students feel comfortable and competent after three hours of practicing it with each other. Anyone who can follow simple instructions can master it.

Self-confidence is the main requirement for practicing Basic ERT with others. I see the quickest self-confidence in those who work one-on-one with people. This includes professionals such as doctors, nurses, teachers, clergymen, psychotherapists, dentists, physical therapists, and massage therapists. But this also includes people who want to help family and friends, parents who nurture their children, spouses who nurture each other, volunteers in churches and the community, people who train and teach others about anything. These people possess "people skills." Their primary motivation is wanting to help others.

With Emotional Release Therapy, we trust people. We trust that they know their emotional pains. Also, in the midst of ERT, the client begins connecting to one emotional pain after another. In this process, clients connect with and release emotions that they did not initially know were there.

So your role as practitioner in Basic ERT with others is limited to telling them to release and then to monitor that release. That is why ERT is so easy to practice.

No self-disclosure or counseling needs to be included with Emotional Release Therapy. If you are a professional psychotherapist, you are welcome to include your therapy along with ERT, but it is unnecessary.

Little information about the ERT client is necessary. I like that! As a pastoral counselor, I know that most people are uncomfortable with sharing their deepest emotional pain. After successfully counseling couples about their marriage, I observed with sadness active members dropping out of the church because I, their pastor, knew the darkest intimate details of their lives.

I know that many people avoid any situation where they have to tell someone the intimate details of their lives. I have no interest in being a voyeur, unnecessarily listening in on the private lives of people. You would be wise to follow this wisdom, too. When you do so, people do not feel threatened by your approach and will trust you to work with them.

You may offer ERT to someone. You need not give ERT a name. Just say, "I have learned a skill that may help you release your emotional pain. Would you be willing to try it?"

You can practice on family members, friends, neighbors, fellow workers, the sick, shut-ins, the recently widowed, and people who are depressed.

For those who come to you and ask for Emotional Release Therapy, ask if they know what they want to release. Most know. If they say yes, I ask them if they would like to talk about it. Most people say no.

A few people will feel a need to tell you all their problems, like they might do in a counseling session. If given the option, some will talk for hours. But after a few minutes with such people, I interrupt, saying something like: "You do not need to tell me all of this. You are telling me your story in an effort to ease your emotional pain. But during Emotional Release Therapy, all your emotional pain will be gone and you will no longer feel this need to tell your story. We have one hour together. We can spend this time getting rid of your emotional pain or I can listen to your story and you can return another time for Emotional Release Therapy. Which do you want to do?" Everyone chooses to move on to the ERT session.

When massage therapist Ken McDonald, quoted in chapter 7, came to me for an Emotional Release Therapy session, I used the basic approach that I am about to teach you. After seeing what it could do, he sponsored an ERT seminar and learned to practice ERT. When I sought testimonials for this book, he immediately provided me with the statement quoted earlier.

With that statement, I learned for the first time that he had released anxiety during our session together. After that session, he had told me he had released what he needed to release. I accepted him at his word. I also learned for the first time about the resolution of his health issues. My approach with ERT does not change, whether the person has health problems or not. I offered Ken Basic ERT and it brought him emotional peace as well as a return to physical health.

Remember that emotional pain is the initial cause of most health problems. Remove the emotional pain with ERT and the cells of the body experience peace. This frees them to regenerate their health.

Most of us are very resourceful at burying emotional pain so deeply that we are unaware of it. This is Nature's way of protecting us from emotional overload. We couldn't bear to be consciously aware of our lifetime of emotional trauma. But we are not home free. Buried emotional pain eventually fills us with anger, fear, anxiety, and depression.

But some emotional traumas are so immense that they daily haunt people. These traumas include childhood and spousal abuse, crime, being the victim of an accident or fire, and the death of loved ones.

For instance, Clara, a 69-year-old woman from Green Bay, Wisconsin, had suffered daily emotional trauma from her rape at age 25. Following 12 minutes of Emotional Release Therapy over the phone, her 44-year nightmare was over and she finally found peace.

New research data on the effects of the mind on the body indicate that emotional pain directly affects recovery from cancer, heart disease, colds, migraine headaches, asthma, ulcers, chronic fatigue, and back pain. When you are emotionally at peace, your body's tendency is to heal itself. I have used ERT on people with all these conditions with success.

ERT can be practiced with infants, children, youths, and adults of all ages. It can also be practiced on animals like dogs, cats, and horses, who seem to be just as vulnerable to emotional trauma as humans. In the following chapters, you will learn to practice ERT on all these beings.

The Practice of ERT

ERT can be practiced in person by touch, in person without touch, and over the phone. ERT without touch and over the phone will be covered in other chapters.

Find a bowl large enough to place your whole hand in it. Put two tablespoons of salt into the bowl and half fill it with hot water. Place the saltwater bowl near where you are going to work along with a towel. A saltwater hand rinse will dissolve the toxic emotions that are about to be released into your hand.

Decide on the position you are going to use so that you can comfortably place your hand on your client's chest for a long period of time without your arm growing tired. The position is described in detail later in this chapter.

The best way is to have your client lie on a massage table or the floor or with loved ones on a bed. Sit beside your client's head. Ask permission to touch your client.

Reach down and place your dominant hand flat on his breastbone (sternum), which is the bony area just above the heart.

Ask the client to close his eyes and you close your own eyes.

Offer a vocal prayer that expresses your intentions.

Ask the client to choose a color and place it in his heart under your hand.

Ask the client to feel the emotions he wishes to release and then to release his feelings into the color in his heart.

Most clients do not feel the heat of their release. So, to know they are releasing, they must depend on your feedback. When you feel the heat of the released feelings begin to enter your hand, you know he is releasing. Let your client know he is releasing and that whatever he is doing, he is doing it right. Say, "You are releasing. You are doing it right."

When your hand grows very warm with the emotional release, dip it into the saltwater bowl to dissolve the toxic emotions that have been released into it. Then dry it with the towel. This dissolves the destructive emotions that have entered your hand as a heat-energy. Return your hand to your client's breastbone.

Keep going through this process until your client is finished releasing his destructive emotions.

With hand in place, offer a vocal prayer blessing. This is a must! People will feel empty after an ERT session. But even more important, during the prayer, you can fill people with personal traits they need. This a powerful tool. A prayer model will be provided. All the prayers are religiously neutral so they can be used with everyone.

Basic ERT is usable when the person can get in touch with all the emotions he needs to release and releases them through the preceding process. This includes destructive emotional states such as anger, fear, anxiety, depression, grief, unhappiness, and worry. It includes painful memories from earlier in life, from loved ones, friends, and work associates, job losses, financial worries, trauma from crime-accident-fire.

Advanced ERT gets to concealed emotions that are not readily accessible by the client. These include destructive emotions from past lives, childhood trauma, sexual abuse, physical abuse, trauma-induced amnesia, post-traumatic stress disorder, anxiety attacks, panic disorders, phobias, obsessive-compulsive behavior, multiple personality disorder, emotionally traumatized body tissue, diseased body tissue, asthma, and allergies.

This biggest obstacle to practicing ERT is that the practitioner's arm can grow heavy and become tired and sore. If right-handed, always sit to the right side of your client, facing his right side (except in position 1, when you are behind and to the left of the client). You will place your right hand flat on the client's breastbone. You will be leaving your hand resting there for up to an hour. So the most difficult part of practicing Emotional Release Therapy is keeping your arm from growing overly tired. Following are some positions for conducting ERT.

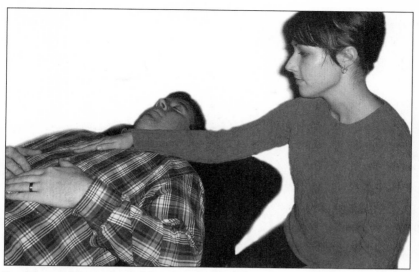

Position 1: Massage Table. This is the easiest position. You can rest your elbow on the table.

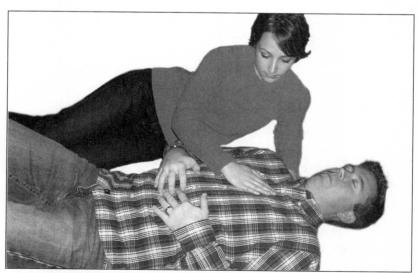

Position 2: Floor or Bed. The second-easiest position. Rest your hand on his chest.

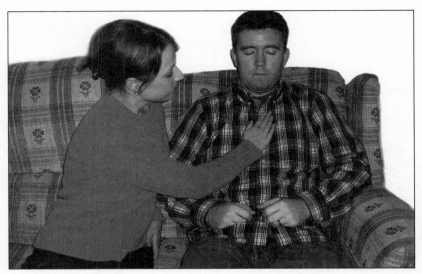

Position 3: Recliner. Recline the client and rest your hand on his chest.

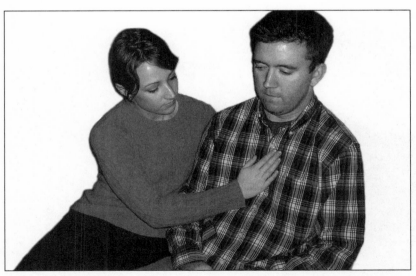

Position 4: Couch or Love Seat. Rest the client against the back cushions and place your hand on his chest.

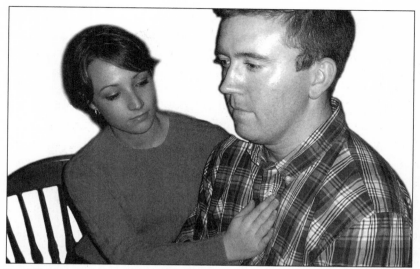

Position 5: Two Straight-Backed Chairs. Use only in training sessions.

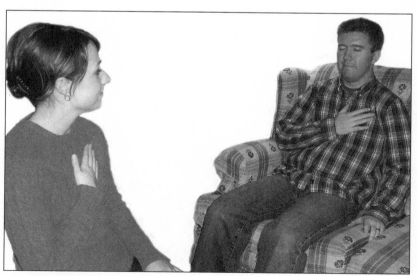

Position 6: Chairs Several Feet Apart. Practice ERT without touching the client. This is only for psychologists or teachers.

Massage Table: With the client lying flat on his back, pull a chair up to his left. Sit by your client's head and reach down with your hand to the client's breastbone. If your chair is the proper height, this is the best way to practice ERT.

Floor or Bed. With loved ones and close friends, you can use a bed or the floor. Lie on your side to the right of the client and rest your right hand on his chest. This position is the easiest on your arm.

Recliner. Use a love seat or couch that has a recliner. Have the client sit in the recliner and recline. This way your hand can rest somewhat effortlessly on the client's chest.

Couch or Love Seat. Use a couch or love seat and sit to the right of the client with your hand on his breastbone. I am tall and am able to rest my elbow on my own thigh when doing this. People come in all heights and shapes, so you must practice to see what works for you. When the sitting position tires your arm, you can stand and do it.

Two Straight-Backed Chairs. Use two straight-backed chairs, and if right-handed, let your chair face the right side of the client. It is helpful to have an armrest on one of the chairs on which you can rest your forearm or elbow. If your arm grows tired, you can stand behind the client and drape your hand onto the breastbone. I use this chair positioning during my seminars, but rarely otherwise.

Chairs Several Feet Apart. Therapists and teachers usually cannot touch their clients and students in such an intimate way so, sitting across a room from each other, they each place their hand on the heart and practice ERT from a distance. This is explained later.

Since practitioners, clients, and chairs come in various heights and shapes, you must experiment to discover the positioning that works best for you. Don't begin practicing ERT until you have discovered the best positioning for you; otherwise the pain in your arm may discourage you from continuing the session.

Protecting Yourself from the Destructive Emotions of Others

Practitioners must protect themselves from taking on the released feelings of emotional pain during ERT, because emotional pain has a life of its own and, when released from the client into your hand, is toxic. So unless you take precautions, you will take on the toxic energy of the emotional pain. For instance, if your client is releasing depression, you can become depressed from the energy of his released depression entering your heart.

Unaware, I practiced ERT with hundreds of clients for two years, storing others' pain in my body. I stored most of the emotional pain in my calves. My calves became so painful that I could hardly walk.

While I was visiting a spiritual master, Babaji, in the Himalayas, a woman told me the cause of my painful calves and how to rid myself of the stored destructive emotions. I followed her directions and it worked. If you use this precaution, you will have no problems.

Solution: A Saltwater Rinse. While practicing ERT, you must rinse your hand in hot saltwater. Before practicing ERT, find a bowl that is large enough to dip your whole hand in. Measure two tablespoons of salt into it and then half fill the bowl with hot water.

When your hand grows warm during ERT, rinse your hand in the hot saltwater, dry it with a dish towel, and return your hand to the client's breastbone. You will be dipping your hand about every two to three minutes. The saltwater dissolves the toxic released emotions. This is the safe way to practice ERT.

Coping with Toxic Emotions of Others on a Daily Basis

If you work directly with people, you are possibly already filled with their emotional pain. This is especially true if you touch people. Everyone emits the energy of their emotions into the people around them. This has happened to you if every evening you are so exhausted that you can hardly function. This is because you are taking in the destructive emotions that other people are emitting and storing them within you.

Walking through a shopping mall for an hour can exhaust some people. Loving, compassionate people share their plentiful energy with people in about a 50-foot radius around them. They also take in other people's negative emotions such as depression, anxiety, anger, and fear.

Solution: A Saltwater Bath. To remove the fatigue you have picked up from others, take a saltwater bath. Almost weekly, I take a saltwater bath. I put six cups of salt in the bathtub and fill it with very warm water.

I then soak for an hour, half while sitting and half lying down, with a saltwater-soaked face cloth over my heart and then on my abdomen. Afterward, I shower off the salt. I always feel lighter, more peaceful, and energized. Why not try this before practicing ERT?

Ken McDonald writes of his first saltwater bath: "The salt bath was incredible! I felt like a foot of fat just fell off me and into the tub. I also did a good ERT release while in the tub of salted water."

Any Salt Will Do. The cheapest salt is Morton's System Saver, a water softener salt found at Kmart or WalMart, and in grocery stores in a 40-pound bag for $4 to $6.

Plastic Wrap. To protect yourself from the negative energy of others, use kitchen plastic wrap. Tear off about 12 inches. Place the plastic wrap on your bare skin on your solar plexus (just below the rib cage). This will protect you from people-derived fatigue all day long. To keep it secure, you might want to wrap it completely around your body. Beware, it can crackle when you move.

Showers. Do not take showers in the morning if you will be with people within an hour after the shower. Showering washes off the body's natural protective layer for about an hour. It would be best to take a shower after coming home for the day. It washes off much of the negative energy you have taken on while being in the world.

Pendants for Protection

Two companies produce a neck pendant that creates a personal shield that protects you from the negative energy of people and the electromagnetic radiation from computer screens, high-power lines, radio and TV signals, and microwave radiation. People wearing these report less stress, more energy and vitality, greater clarity and focus, and emotional balance.

The Q-Link Pendant: Developed by energy medicine researchers at the University of California at Los Angeles, it contains a computer chip charged by the body's energy. It is put out by Clarus Products (www.qlinkproducts.com) and costs $129.

The BioElectric Shield: This pendant containing crystal and copper costs $139, but comes with a discount coupon for a second one at $20 off (www.bioelectriccompany.com).

Why Use a Color?

The ERT direction is: "Choose a color and place it under the hand on your chest." Why do you need to focus on a color? It is easier to release your fleeting feelings into a concrete image than into nothing but a vague space. The color you choose does not matter. If during the ERT process the color changes, tell your client to use the new one.

Maintaining a color is easier if you do not try hard. Just casually let the color be there. As you practice ERT, the color stabilizes. The color is not the only possible focus. You can make the color into a river or waterfall, through which your feelings can flow into the hand on your chest.

Some people are unable to imagine a color. In that case, the feelings can be released directly into the hand. If this does not work, clients can talk about their emotional pain while doing ERT, though this takes longer to do.

One Must Release Emotions

One must release *emotions,* not *thoughts.* It is emotions, not thoughts, that are painful. Releasing thoughts about emotions does not work. You must tell your clients to release the feelings of their emotional pain, not their thoughts. Released thoughts produce a sensation of tingling, not heat. Your clients' ability to feel emotions determines the ease with which they release their emotional pain.

Tell your clients to release what they are feeling as the ERT session begins. Once they begin releasing one emotion, they will enter an emotional state of consciousness that helps them connect to one emotion after another. Once that begins, they may go on for as much as an hour of effortless release. When they finish, they may feel exhausted but will feel at peace.

At times, a client's mind may wander as she mentally searches for what to release next. Even then, she may still be releasing her feelings. The hand on her chest will know this.

Children are the best at release. Some are able to release all their emotional pain within ten minutes. Those who have experienced considerable emotional pain may take as long as an adult. Even thinking types release well once they shift into their emotional consciousness.

Monitoring the Emotional Release of Others

Those releasing are usually unaware of their release within themselves. It is the hand on the breastbone that feels the emotional release as heat energy. It is this hand that must monitor the release through its sensing of the heat of the released emotions. When that begins to happen, you tell the client, "You are now releasing your emotions. Just keep on doing what you are doing because it is working." Your hand will grow warmer and warmer as it fills with the heat of the releasing emotions. As it does, you lose your ability to feel the heat release.

Rinsing your hand in the saltwater removes the heat in your hand and renews your hand's sensing ability. When you place your rinsed hand back on the breastbone, if you still feel heat, provide more feedback to the client by saying, "You are still releasing."

If, when waiting for the release to begin, you feel a tingling instead of heat, your client is releasing thoughts, not feelings. Tell the client, "Focus upon releasing feelings, not thoughts." Most will quickly begin releasing the heat of their emotions.

There is an exception to this rule. The released emotions of children aged 12 and under often feel like a tingle or energy. I think this is due to their immense youthful energy.

Not All Clients Are Releasing

If the client states he cannot get in touch with his feelings, tell him to release feelings, not thoughts. If this does not work, keep your hand in place and suggest that he talk about his emotional pain.

Tell him to keep his eyes shut. Let him know when he begins releasing heat into your hand. Ask him to try again to release silently. If this does not work, go through the session letting him talk.

A very few people will not be able to release. When this happens, take a five-minute break. Then try again. This usually works. If this doesn't work, make another appointment. At the next session, I guarantee the client will have figured out how to do it.

When the Practitioner Cannot Feel Release

Some practitioners are unable to feel heat entering their hands, even though the client states he is releasing his emotional pain. To check on his progress, ask, "Is the emotion you are releasing declining in strength?"

If the client says yes, he is releasing into your hand, but you cannot sense it. Don't be discouraged. Let the client monitor his own release. Tell him that when he no longer feels the emotion, it is gone. Ask him then to proceed to another emotion. In this way, you can be just as effective.

During a workshop, one of my students could not feel any heat release. But from the feedback of others she practiced with at the seminar, it was obvious that she was being effective. A week after her seminar, she told me she had successfully practiced ERT with seven people. She did this by having her own unique awareness of the released emotions. She could not describe this awareness. She just knew. I reminded her that, even though she wasn't feeling the heat, she still had to rinse her hand periodically in saltwater.

10

Practicing Emotional Release Therapy with Others

The technique in this chapter is similar to self-healing Basic ERT and Advanced ERT. Before proceeding, you need to review the previous chapter.

Here you learn to practice Emotional Release Therapy with others. This is rewarding work. Before your eyes, you see the immediate results. People come to you in emotional pain and leave at peace. Often you are amazed with the results. Never before have you helped people so easily and so substantially. It builds your self-confidence and self-respect. The practical help you render may fascinate you.

During and after ERT, you will likely feel serenity. It may be a spiritual experience that centers you in God. About ten percent of the time, both you and your client enter a state of bliss, which can last for 15 to 30 minutes after the session.

Practicing ERT with others also makes you comfortable with practicing physical healing. In physical healing, you follow similar processes but seldom see immediate results. With ERT, you follow the process and see the immediate results. You know the ERT process works, so you grow comfortable with the physical healing techniques you are using. This enables you to become confident in practicing physical healing.

Some find life fulfillment in ERT. As Marlene explains, "It has changed my whole life and I can now use the talents I have known I have had for a long time."

Instructions for Practicing ERT with Others

Saltwater. Before your client arrives, put two tablespoons of salt into a bowl. Half fill the bowl with hot water when you are ready to use it, but not before. Otherwise the water will become uncomfortably cool halfway into your session. Obtain a towel to dry your hand.

Prepare the place where you are going to work. Plan where to place your client and yourself. Make sure your needed posture will not tire your arm. The room should be quiet and at a comfortable temperature. Noise from other rooms should be minimized. If you like to work with music in the background, prepare this. Artificial lighting should be adjusted to the subdued mode for the session.

Who should be present? I prefer to be alone with my clients. This way the energy in the room is only you and your client. The exception is having a parent present if child clients are fearful. Have another adult present if there might be suspicions of sexual overtones between you and the client. Sometimes a spouse wants to stay while you are working with the other spouse. I try to discourage this but sometimes find myself stuck.

Greeting the client. Go through all of a host's normal social amenities. Initially, let the client sit anyplace. Get his or her name, address, phone number, and, if possible, e-mail address.

Explain in your own words how ERT works. Tell your client that no self-disclosure is necessary. Ask if your client knows what he or she needs to release. If there is hesitation, let the client talk about it, but briefly.

After five minutes or so, say, "You seem to now know what you need to release. I suggest the best use of our time now is to begin Emotional Release Therapy. After Emotional Release Therapy, you will not feel the need to tell me your story."

Immediate preparation. Show the client where to lie or sit during ERT. Excuse yourself to half fill the saltwater bowl with hot water. Place the bowl and towel within easy reach of where you will be. Take your positions.

Beginning ERT. Ask the client, "May I place my hand on your breastbone?" As you say this, place your hand upon your own breastbone to model what you are about to do. Place your hand flat on the client's breastbone.

Direct the client. Say, "Let us close our eyes throughout the session." Close your eyes, too. "Let us pray. God, help _____ [client's name] get in touch with his/her emotional pain and release those feelings into my hand. Help me receive them in love. Thank you, God. Amen."

ERT instructions. Say to the client, "Now, I want you to place a color under my hand and begin releasing the feelings of the emotions you wish to release into the color and into my hand. I can feel your release in my hand and will tell you when you are releasing."

Coaching. Focus upon your hand. When you feel heat begin to enter it, inform the client, "You are releasing. Whatever you are doing, continue doing because it is working." It is unusual for a client not to release his or her emotions into your hand.

Feeling tingling. If you feel a tingling, the client is releasing thoughts. Say, "You are releasing thoughts. Try to release feelings." Usually, this works and you begin feeling a heat release. The client already knows how to release, so shifting to a feeling release is fairly simple.

Feeling nothing. If you feel nothing entering your hand, this means one of two things. Usually, it means the client is not releasing. Encouragingly, say, "Release your feelings, not your thoughts."

If this does not work, ask, "Is your emotional pain diminishing?" If the client says yes, the client is releasing, but you are not feeling it. This means you will have to let the client monitor his or her own release. Say, "Just keep releasing. When you no longer feel an emotion, it is gone and you can move on to another emotion."

Or the client will say, "I can't hold the color." If so, say, "Forget the color. Just release your feelings directly into my hand."

Or the client will say, "I can't get in touch with my emotions." If so, say, "Keep your eyes closed and tell me what you wish to release." As the client talks, he or she should begin releasing.

If none of this works, take a break or schedule another appointment.

In doing so, the client usually figures out how to release his or her emotions.

Your inner life. Initially focus on your hand as you wait to feel the release. Sometimes I imagine my hand is a magnet, drawing the client's emotions into it. I have had a few clients tell me afterward that they felt no release, though I sensed intense release. Perhaps I was pulling the emotions out of the person. Sometimes I silently pray for the client. Sometimes my mind is blank or wandering. Regardless of what you are doing, release occurs. I think that once you state your intentions, the process continues with your hand receiving the release.

Rinse often in saltwater. When your hand grows very warm with accumulated emotions or after three minutes of release with no sense of a heat release, rinse your hand in the saltwater bowl, towel it dry, and place it again on the client's breastbone. The saltwater dissolves the still alive released emotion. If the heat begins moving up your arm, use the other hand to brush it back down into your hand. This is a warning to rinse more often. Rinsing your hand also makes your hand more sensitive to feeling the emotional release.

Feeling nothing temporarily. It is not unusual for the heat release to stop for a while. If it does, remind the client, "Release your feelings." The releasing may have stopped because the client is thinking of what to release next or his or her mind has wandered.

When the client finishes. Clients often don't tell you when they are finished. After your client has released for a long time and the release stops, ask, "Are you finished?" The client may say no, and you continue. But usually he or she says, "I think so" or "Yes." Now you begin to guide the client.

Go to the abdomen. Ask permission, as in, "May I place my hand on your abdomen?" Slowly move your flattened hand to the client's abdomen. Tell your client to place the color under your hand and ask him or her to release feelings down there into your hand. Again, inform the client when releasing has begun. Let him or her release as long as needed. If you feel no release, no emotions are stored there. Rinse your hand often.

Go to the solar plexus. Ask permission, saying, "May I place my hand on your solar plexus?" Move your hand to the client's solar plexus (just below the ribs). Rarely will you feel a release, but do it anyway, just in case. Rinse your hand often.

Emotional pain from loved ones. Explain to the client, "The people who can wound us the worst are our loved ones and people at work. Let's begin with your grandmothers, whether dead or alive. If there is anything about your paternal grandmother that annoys you or has hurt you or disappointed you, release your feelings into my hand."

Rinse your hand often. When the heat stops for a while, ask, "Are you finished?"

Continue with the client's maternal grandmother.

Then move on to the grandfathers, saying, "If there is anything about your paternal grandfather that annoys you or has hurt you or disappointed you, release your feelings into my hand." Rinse your hand often. When the heat stops for a while, ask, "Are you finished?"

Continue with the maternal grandfather.

Then move on to the client's father, saying, "If there is anything about your father that annoys you or has hurt you or disappointed you, release your feelings into my hand." Rinse your hand often. When the heat stops for a while, ask, "Are you finished?"

Then go to mother, spouse or lover, children, siblings.

Go to any other family members who have affected the client. Go to friends individually. Go to the workplace and release difficulties at work and relational problems with other persons.

Improving self-image. Explain, "What keeps you from looking in the mirror and saying, I am OK in every way? This exercise is about releasing negative self-images. Is there anything about yourself you do not like, like your physical appearance, personality, character, inadequacy, shame, embarrassment, guilt? Release your feelings about each of these into my hand." Afterward, rinse your hand.

Hidden emotional pain from gestation, birth, and early childhood. Explain, "Now let's go to your unremembered painful emotions while you were in your mother's womb. When I count to one, release any emotional pain that was inflicted on you from the moment of your conception to your birth. 3, 2, 1, release."

If you feel a strong release, repeat this exercise. Afterward, rinse your hand. Now go with birth, then ages one, two, three, four, five, and six, and do the same thing: "When I count to one, release any emotional pain that was inflicted on you from the moment of your birth to age one . . . 3, 2, 1, release."

Hidden emotional pain from childhood. Explain, "Now let's go to your later childhood's unremembered painful emotions. When I count to one, release any emotional pain that was inflicted on you at age six . . . 3, 2, 1, release." If you feel a strong release, repeat this exercise. Afterward, rinse your hand.

Now go to ages seven, eight, nine, ten, 11, and 12. Do each age individually.

Hidden emotional pain from youth. Explain, "Now let's go to your youth and unremembered painful emotions. When I count to one, release any emotional pain that was inflicted on you at age 13 . . . 3, 2, 1, release."

If you feel a strong release, repeat this exercise. Afterward, rinse your hand.

Now go to ages 14, 15, 16, 17, 18, and 19, individually.

Hidden emotional pain from adulthood. Explain, "Now you are going to release emotional pain that you have deeply buried from age 20 to 30. When I count to one, you will release any emotional pain that you suffered from ages 20 to 30 . . . 3, 2, 1, release." There may be a delay in feeling the release, so be patient.

If you feel a strong release, repeat this exercise. Rinse your hand as needed.

Continue on with each decade in turn: 30–40, 40–50, and so forth.

Past emotional pain. Return your hand to the breastbone. Tell the client, "You are now going to release emotional pain from throughout your life. Go back through every painful time and release the emotional trauma of it. Every hurt you have ever known is still stored someplace in your heart. Recall moments of rejection, blame, shame, embarrassment, grief, failure, guilt, and broken relationships. If you cannot feel it, try to relive it and imagine what your emotions would have been. Release the emotional pain of every such memory as a feeling into my hand. Tell me when you are done."

Rinse your hand often. When the release stops for a while, ask, "Are you finished?"

Cutting ties. Explain, "If you have people in your past or present who haunt you with painful emotions, you probably have a cord of energy binding you to them. This energy bond may be with an estranged or deceased spouse or lover, parent, child, sibling, friend, coworker, or whomever. Cutting your energy ties to them can stop your emotional discomfort and give you a new sense of freedom. Do this exercise one person at a time.

"Visualize a cord of energy connecting you to him or her. Then take an imaginary pair of scissors and cut this connecting cord to sever any energy contact with that person. While you do this, I will pray for you."

While the client works at this, pray aloud, "God, I cut this cord that binds _____ [client's name] to this person. May the bond between them be completely severed that _____ [client's name] might be at peace with him or her. Thank you. Amen." Afterward, rinse your hand.

Past lives. Explain, "Past lives is a term referring to previous lives that your soul has experienced in other physical identities of which you have no memory. Some people believe that the trauma and sin (karmic debt) in your past lives harmfully influence your present life. Whether or not you believe in past lives, let's see what might be there."

"When I count to one, release all the past-life pain that is harming your life today . . . 3, 2, 1, release." If you feel a strong release, repeat this exercise. Rinse your hand as needed.

The Prayer Blessing

Having finished Emotional Release Therapy, you must fill the client with a prayer blessing. Say that you usually bless the client with love and peace. Ask what other qualities the client would like to add. Usually, there is nothing. But if there is, add it to your prayer blessing. Here is a prayer model: "God, fill _____ [client's name] with love and peace and _____ [add whatever they have suggested]. Thank you. Amen."

This completes the instructions for practicing ERT with others.

Now, run through the instructions again. Find a family member or friend and run through it several times with various persons. Get their feedback. Finding clients who need ERT is your next challenge. If you are a professional, you may have ready-made clients.

If you belong to a group of some sort, let it be known that you have skills that heal emotional pain. You can design a flyer and post it in your neighborhood or apartment complex. The next few chapters give you clues about how others found clients.

11

Practicing ERT BodyTalk for Physical Healing

A woman phoned me. Her husband had colon cancer that had spread to his liver and he had only days to live. Could I help him? I inwardly groaned. Why am I the last resort? Why don't people contact me in the early stages of disease? I knew there was only about a 50 percent of healing Howard at this stage of the disease. I answered, "I don't know. It all depends on how well Howard cooperates. Have him phone me."

Sixty-seven-year-old Howard phoned me from his Oklahoma home. He sounded sick and prepared to die, a reluctant healee whom I had agreed to pull from death's door.

That week we had three phone sessions that involved ERT and ERT BodyTalk. Even though I was not optimistic about his recovery, I followed the processes fully.

Howard surprised me by cooperating well. By the third session, he stated that he was feeling better. He was eating well and no longer slept 14 hours a day. He was taking daily walks and he intended to return to his office two days a week. Two weeks later, his wife sent me a check for my

services with a note. It read that Howard was practicing ERT and ERT BodyTalk on himself and he felt well. Two weeks later, Howard phoned me. He had just had an MRI and was cancer free.

I asked him why he had waited so long to call me. He said he didn't believe in such things until he was so sick that he thought he would die. Only then had his wife called me in desperation.

Spiritual healing remains one of the most misunderstood, unbelieved, ridiculed, and shunned subjects in the world. I am hoping that my rational explanation of healing helps to change all of this.

The fear, anger, shame, and embarrassment that have always surrounded healing have never prevented healers from healing. Throughout the centuries, intuitive, creative, compassionate persons have always found themselves being drawn to practice healing, initially almost against their will. They want to be accepted by people and healing only leads to rejection.

Eventually, they find joy and fulfillment in healing. It is as though they are finally home and are fulfilling their soul's longing. They become fascinated by everything there is to know about healing. Healing encounters fill them with spiritual bliss.

Now, you have read most of this book. You have tried the exercises. You have experienced the practice of healing. What is your response to this book?

A person can store emotional and physical trauma in every cell of the body. This is true of people with chronic and life-threatening conditions such as chronic fatigue syndrome, fibromyalgia, multiple sclerosis, muscular dystrophy, Lou Gehrig's disease, and cancer. They are supersaturated with emotional and physical trauma in every cell of their body. Using ERT BodyTalk, talk to a person's body and it will release all the trauma it holds.

All diseases leave their trauma in the body. If you suffered a heart attack, stroke, or cancer 20 years ago, the cells remember the agony of the disease and of the treatment. With ERT BodyTalk, the body will release trauma from diseases it had many years ago. ERT BodyTalk is the best physical healing method that I have used.

ERT must always precede BodyTalk. It may take two or more sessions of ERT to remove all the emotional pain. Keep using ERT until the person is at emotional peace. If you can teach others to do ERT on themselves, they can effectively practice it daily.

Practice ERT! Practice ERT BodyTalk! They always work! They always bring people back to health! Follow the process and see the blessed results. Emotional pain causes the healing frequency to be distorted so that it can't heal. In fact, emotional pain keeps people from healing with medical care. With ERT BodyTalk, you will fill your client's whole body with God's healing power.

Using BodyTalk with One or Two Medical Conditions

You can do this on a person who has one or two medical conditions. For instance, if a woman has a bladder infection, with your hand on her heart, talk to the bladder. Say, "Bladder, release your emotional pain and your dysfunction into my hand on my heart. Also, release the pain surrounding you."

When the heat stops entering your hand, rinse your hand in saltwater. If the release is strong, repeat this procedure.

Then place your hand on top of her head. Say something like this: "God, send your healing power into her brain. Brain, open a door and let the healing power in. Let it flow throughout you, brain, healing all your functions.

"Now let the healing power flow down through the torso and into the bladder. Heal the bladder. Restore every cell in the bladder to normal and make the bladder healthy and whole. Heal the surrounding tissue of the bladder. Recreate and make all tissue new and normal. Thank you for the healing that is taking place."

Leave your hand on top of her head for ten minutes. Do this for three days. Her bladder may be healed on the first or second day, but you are taking precautions and doing it for three days.

Hand position. Place your dominant hand on your client's heart. Close your eyes.

Talk to the body one organ/part at a time. Say, "Brain, release your emotional pain, your physical discomfort, and your dysfunction into my hand when I count to one. 3, 2, 1, release." The release is delayed compared to ERT. If the release is strong, repeat the procedure. Do this with the brain, ears, eyes, sinuses, nose, throat, lungs, heart, liver, pancreas, spleen, esophagus, stomach, intestines, bladder, reproductive organs, sex organs, kidneys, nervous system, muscles, bone joints, blood vessels, blood, skin, and so forth. Rinse your hand often in the saltwater.

Say, "_____ [name the body part], release your emotional pain, your physical discomfort, and your dysfunction into my hand. 3, 2, 1, release."

Filling the Body with God's Healing Power

Hand position. You and your client both close your eyes. Now change your hand position on your client. Place your dominant hand on top of your client's head.

Pray. "God, may your healing power flow from my hand into his/her brain. Thank you. Amen."

Talk to the brain. Say to the brain, "Brain, open a door and let this healing flow in." Mentally visualize it flowing into your client's brain.

Talk to God. "God's healing power, flow throughout her brain, restoring all brain functions, and fill them with your healing and peace. Amen." Imagine it flowing throughout your client's brain.

Now, do the same thing with the body's organs and parts. These include the eyes, ears, sinuses, nose, mouth, throat, lungs, heart, liver, gallbladder, pancreas, spleen, esophagus, stomach, intestines, bladder, kidneys, reproductive organs, sexual organs, nerves, muscles, bone joints, blood vessels, blood, skin, and so forth.

With your dominant hand on top of your client's head, pray: "God, may your healing power flow from my hand into his/her _____ [body part]. God's healing power, flow throughout his/her ____ [body part], restoring her health and wholeness and filling her with your peace. Amen." Imagine it flowing throughout that body part or organ.

Healing Body Sections

Place your hand on the top of your client's head and pray, "God, may your healing power flow from my hand into her brain, renewing every cell in her head, flow down her right arm into her fingers, renewing every cell in her right arm, flow down her left arm into her fingers, renewing every cell in her right arm, flow from her brain down her throat into the whole torso, renewing every cell in her torso, flow down her right leg to her toes, renewing every cell in her right leg, flow down her left leg to her toes, renewing every cell in her left leg. Flow throughout her body, healing her and filling her with peace. Amen."

This completes ERT BodyTalk. We now go on to other forms of physical healing.

Charged Towel

For selective body healing, charge a cotton dish towel with the healing energy. Fold the towel and hold it between your hands. Pray, "God, fill this towel with your healing power that it might heal her. Thank you. Amen." Charge the towel in your hands for about 15 minutes. While charging it, you can talk, watch TV, or read. Fold the towel to the desired size. Have your client place it on her bare skin at the intended area. Have her secure it with her clothing or, if the area is on a limb, have her use rubber bands loosely around it to hold it in place. Let it remain there 24 hours a day. It is releasing a healing energy, like an IV gives your body healing substances. Your client will know it is working by the slight heat she will feel under the towel. The towel loses its healing energy as it heals. Recharge it once a week.

I have successfully used this with trauma injuries, arthritis, angina, diseased organs, skin diseases, surgical wounds, sore throats, sinus infections, and sunburn.

Energized Water

You can charge water with healing energy, just as you did a towel. Hold a gallon jug or other water container in both hands. Pray, "God, fill this water with your healing power so that the water will heal her body. Thank you. Amen." Hold it for 15 minutes. While holding it, you can talk, watch TV, or read. Your hands know what to do and need no further effort on your part. Have your client drink two ounces of the healing charged water with every meal and at bedtime. The water will release healing energy into every cell.

Repeat this process several times daily until three days after all symptoms are gone.

Localized Conditions

If the condition is due to an injury, surgery, or a disease present in one location in the body, use the following process. The sooner you practice healing on a trauma injury, the more quickly symptoms disappear. An immediately treated sprained ankle will have no symptoms within five minutes. Deep auto accident bruises on the thigh can be gone in a day.

Remove the trauma. Place your dominant hand about one-quarter inch above the skin. Talk to that location, saying something like, "Release your emotional pain, your physical discomfort, and your confusion into my hand." You may or may not feel the heat of the release. Hold your hand there for about a minute. Then either shake your hand to rid yourself of the body's release or dip it in a bowl of saltwater.

Practice healing. Place your hand on the skin. If the location is on an arm or a leg, use both hands, one on either side. Offer a prayer, like, "God, may your healing power flow through my hand(s) and into her body. Make every cell normal and fill them with your peace. Thank you. Amen." Hold your hand(s) there for about a minute.

Open the body. After the prayer, talk to her body. Say, "Open a door under my hand and let the healing flow in." Sometimes you will feel her body's immediate intake of the healing energy. This can feel like a whoosh, as the body sucks it in.

Assess. Remove your hand(s) and shake it. Then return your hand(s) to the area. If the skin remains cool, the tissue has been filled with all the healing flow it needs and you are finished with this session. If the skin grows warm, more healing energy is needed and keep your hand(s) there for another two minutes. Check your progress again by shaking your hand and replacing it to assess the need. You are now finished with this phase of healing.

Repeat. Do this process twice a day until all the symptoms are gone. You have now completed every form of physical healing.

12

A Working Model for Healing

Our working model for healing begins with the nature of the universe. The universe is composed of matter and energy. Measurable energy fields permeate all matter, including plants, animals, and humans. The human body is interpenetrated by at least seven energy fields, each operating at a different electromagnetic frequency. They radiate from the body at a range from a quarter-inch to more than 25 feet beyond the skin.

The human energy fields contain information, act purposefully, and are essential for life. They duplicate the biological, mental, emotional, and spiritual components of human beings and interact with them. Every human function has its counterpart in the energy fields.

At the lowest frequency of human energy fields, every cell of the physical body is duplicated. Russian researchers state that this energy field is a blueprint for the physical body. Each physical organ is formed and sustained by the blueprint energy field. If the energy mold is misshapen, the product of that mold will be misshapen (and ill) in the same way. Energy fields shape the physical body the way a gelatin mold shapes gelatin. They also interact with the physical body, affecting the blueprint energy field.

This was scientifically proven by the research of Dr. Ramesh Chouhan at the Jipmer regional government hospital in Pondicherry, India, in the 1980s. For eight years, under a grant from the government of India, Dr. Chouhan and his staff screened 25,000 women entering the obstetrical-gynecological (OB-GYN) unit. They took bioelectrographic pictures (an advanced form of Kirlian photography) of the fingertips of patients. Through a massive database of these pictures along with the women's medical histories, Dr. Chouhan discovered the signatures in their energy fields that were predictive of oncoming cancer and arthritis.

The Chouhan scientific research indicates that three to six months before the onset of cancer, the blueprint human energy field becomes distorted in a distinct way that is predictive of the cancer. He discovered energy field distortions six to 12 months before the onset of arthritis.

When I read Dr. Chouhan's research paper in 1987, I asked myself, what could be causing these energy field distortions? Then I remembered several earlier studies by American psychologists that some cancer patients had suffered an emotional trauma about 18 months before the onset of their cancer. I wondered: Could there be a connection between emotional pain and the appearance of the distorted energy fields that were predictive of the onset of cancer and arthritis?

In 1989, I joined Dr. Chouhan in India for further research. Running a low-voltage energy through a person's fingers and using a low-light video camera in the dark, we were able to videotape the changes in the human energy field during my prayer healing sessions with patients. We discovered that patients whose energy fields tested positive for the onset of cancer could have their energy fields returned to normal through healing prayer sessions. These women did not get cancer. This is healing that prevents an expected disease from occurring.

In 1994, a primary care physician referred a late-stage colon cancer patient to me. The Cleveland Clinic had just informed the woman, Maggie, 49, that there was nothing more they could do medically to help her. Maggie and I had two Emotional Release Therapy sessions together, after which Maggie said she was emotionally peaceful and was the happiest she had been since her youth. Six weeks later, Maggie had an MRI (magnetic resonance imaging) that indicated her cancer cells had become normal. She no longer had cancer.

Since then, I have assumed that patients have a unique disease signature in their energy field that either precedes or maintains the diseased condition. With the 1994 discovery of Emotional Release Therapy, I had a new tool to test out that assumption. So far that assumption has been proven valid. I discovered that in most of the people who released their emotional pain, their cancer symptoms disappeared within six weeks. If you follow ERT with touch-healing prayer sessions, the healing outcomes reach almost one hundred percent for specific medical conditions.

Medical research already indicates that stress directly affects recovery from cancer, heart disease, colds, migraine headaches, asthma, ulcers, chronic fatigue, and back pain. I equate stress with emotional pain. I have observed all of these medical conditions being healed after ERT and sometimes with the addition of spiritual healing.

My students and clients have testified to the emotional healing/resolution of the following conditions after ERT alone: academic failure, attention-deficit/hyperactivity disorder (ADHD), agoraphobia, anxiety, bed-wetting, behavioral problems in children and youth, depression, fear, grief, emotional upsets in infant and child, marital unhappiness, panic attacks, post-traumatic stress disorder, resentment, childhood sexual abuse and physical torture, crime victim trauma, trichotillomania, obesity (weight loss of up to 80 pounds), and phobias with snakes, elevators, and storms.

They have also testified to the physical healing, with the use of ERT alone, of allergies, arthritis, asthma, bronchitis, cancer, carpal tunnel syndrome, chronic fatigue syndrome, coughing, fibromyalgia, gluten intolerance, gout, dead muscle from a heart attack, liver disease, liver failure, muscular dystrophy, neck and back pain, and sinusitis.

ERT can also resolve the problems of shyness and talking too much in class. ERT used on fear of poor sports performance can help students in physical education classes. ERT removes blocks to learning certain subjects such as math, which can be of obvious benefit to many students.

Families have many issues that may be helped by ERT. Diaper rash. Aversion to physical exercise. Not wanting to do homework. Weight loss. Conflicts between family members. Anger. Fear. Anxiety. Unhappiness. Depression. Pedophilia.

ERT can change attitudes that are important elements of poverty, juvenile delinquency, criminal behavior, tobacco use, alcohol and drug use, and shoplifting.

Compulsive behavior is caused by possession of the emotions causing the compulsion. ERT should eliminate pedophilia, males exposing themselves, rape, destructive sexual behaviors, and many other behaviors.

If we could identify the specific emotions that trigger a specific disease, ERT is likely to prevent or cure many diseases. Can it consistently cure muscular dystrophy as it did with Justin Thomson, whom you read about in chapter 3? Can it heal Lou Gehrig's disease? Can it heal mental retardation in infants? We don't know and won't know until knowledgeable people try to heal such conditions.

When I lecture or lead a workshop, I begin by asking the audience, "How many of you have lower back pain right now?" Usually, about half raise their hands. Then I demonstrate healing the back through ERT with a volunteer. I ask those who do not have back pain to practice ERT with those who do have back pain. An hour later, I ask how many are free of back pain. Almost everyone is. It is a very convincing demonstration that lower back pain is usually caused by storing emotional pain in the lower back. We can store emotional pain in the lower back, in the neck and shoulders, in the bone joints, in the hands, and in the feet. Women also store emotional pain in the female organs. So you go to the doctor complaining about pain in your body, but the doctor can find nothing wrong. Before consulting a physician, try practicing ERT in the painful area.

A New Way to Restore Health

Traditional spiritual healing was always frustrating for me. When I first discovered in 1966 that I had a gift for healing, I only knew that sometimes healing occurred when I, as a pastor, held the hand of the sick and praying. It was hit or miss.

The only time I knew it was a hit was when the patient or the patient's family, in the next day or two, reported a dramatic recovery. I probably prayed for the healing of more than ten thousand people in my years in the parish ministry.

I did not look for religious and biblical answers to healing. From the beginning, I sought a rational understanding: some sort of a cause-and-effect relationship. It was a lonely journey. At that time, my own Christian tradition and most people considered healing a mystery. We pray for the sick and God mysteriously determines whether our prayers are answered.

I repeatedly heard from others that "God heals and he does it any way he chooses to do it." Or worse, "God chooses to heal some and to let others die."

My response to these beliefs was like Scrooge: "Bah, humbug!" My own belief was that God wants everyone to become well and be healthy. The failure of healing prayer was therefore due to our own ignorance of how prayer works. At that time and to this day, that was considered blasphemy—a profane belief about how God works.

It has been an agonizing, yet joyful journey of rational discovery. I am an observer of healing and have a rational and spiritual understanding. I am a pragmatist and inventor. I believe that if it works, use it. When I have an intuitive insight, I experiment to see if it consistently works for me and for everyone else.

That is the basis for all objective research. I earned a doctorate in healing research in Montreal with biology researcher Bernard Grad, known as the father of healing research, as my faculty advisor. I ask you to join me in trusting practical truths. My words are only true if it works for you. Relax! Be skeptical! Experiment! Yes, this is a serious pursuit for you.

I've been to the drawing board many times. I think I've worked out most of the glitches. Enjoy your journey back to health. You are about to have a fantastic adventure. Savor it!

Given all these rational, practical words, am I actually a religious person? I am a clergyman, grounded in the Christian faith. I cannot remember when I have not felt close to God. God's presence and creative flow are helping to write this book.

Conventional medical care is an excellent option for many conditions. I have immense respect and affection for my primary care physician. He nurtured me back to health in intensive care after food poisoning. I take herbs to lower my cholesterol. I have had my cataracts surgically removed after various alternative approaches failed. My wife and I have annual medical examinations. In fact, I have far more respect for conventional medicine than they have for me. While I believe that what I teach will enhance most medical procedures, doctors don't. Part of this is disbelief, but part of it is protecting their territory.

Healers and scientific researchers, all specialists in the field of healing, believe that God does not directly heal human beings. God uses human agents to do his healing work. Humans attune the healing flow by their love and transmit it to the ill.

Rather than referring to God's healing power or healing flow, scientists use more objective scientific terms. God's healing power becomes an energy that is healing or a healing energy.

Bernard Grad, retired researcher from McGill University, conducted over two hundred studies on the effects of healing touch on plants and animals. He chose these subjects to rule out the placebo factor that would be present when healing humans.

Dr. Grad described healing energy in this way: "The healing energy is informational. The energy itself is an information-bearer, self-regulating, programmed. Where healing calls for the slowing down of cell growth . . . development is inhibited. Where healing requires the speeding up of cell growth . . . the process is accelerated. Slow down or speed up for healing? The same agent does both. The energy itself knows."

More than a thousand studies have provided us with a helpful new picture that makes healing more effective. When scientists study this, they do so from an objective, nonreligious viewpoint. Here is a small portion of the scientific picture.

Infrared shows changes in healer-charged water. A 1986 study by Swartz, Brame, and Spottiswood, "Infrared Spectra Alteration in Water Proximate to Palms of Therapeutic Practitioners" (The Mobius Society, 4801 Wilshire Blvd., Suite 120, Los Angeles, CA 90010), examined the infrared absorption spectra of water placed in sealed vials and treated by 14 different healers. Statistically significant differences in patterns in infrared spectrophotometric analysis were observed between healer-treated water and normal water. An energy had to be emitted to produce the changes in the healer-treated water.

Healer-charged bottled water makes wounded barley seeds grow. Bernard Grad had healer Oskar Estebany hold bottled water while emitting healing energy with his hands. The water was then used for Dr. Grad's Wounded Barley Seed Experiment. The healer-charged water caused barley seeds watered with a one-percent saline solution to grow faster than the controls watered with an untreated one-percent saline solution.

Robert Miller of Atlanta discovered similar growth in plants treated with healer-charged water. This was reported in *Future Science: Life Energies and the Physics of Paranormal Phenomena*, edited by John White and Stanley Krippner (Anchor Books, 1977).

Healer-charged water not diminished in storage. Dr. Grad stored healer-charged water adjacent to untreated water in a dark closet for two years. The healer treated water did not diminish in strength after two years and did not contaminate the adjacent bottled water. This is a unique form of energy.

Healer-charged cotton and wool. In a similar study, healer Oskar Estebany imparted healing energy into cotton and wool cuttings that were placed in induced-goiter-in-mouse cages, preventing the mice from getting goiters, the same effect the healers had.

Healer-charged surgical gauze. Dr. Dolores Krieger reports similar healing results with healer-treated gauze. Applied as a wound dressing, it resulted in faster healing (reported in *Therapeutic Touch,* by Dolores Krieger [Prentice-Hall, 1979]).

Naval physicists found frequencies that induce and heal cancer. Seven U.S. Navy physicists discovered that when a healer placed his hands in water, the water protons began emitting an 8 hertz frequency. They then radiated mice with a 5.xxx hertz frequency, inducing cancer in them within 48 hours. (The "5.xxx frequency" is not named because it could be used in an energy generator placed under a bed to kill people.) When the mice were radiated with the healer frequency of 8 hertz, the mice's tumors were healed within 48 hours. This was published in *Subtle Energies* in 1991.

Life energy produces the optimum conditions for life. A bean experiment by Spindrift, founded by a group of Christian Science practitioners in Salem, Oregon, graphically proved that prayer produces the optimum conditions for life. Three trays were prepared: one with dried-out beans, one with water-soaked beans, and a third with normal beans. In a series of runs, people prayed for the beans. In every case, the three trays ended up with normal beans. The prayers brought normal health to the beans.

Healing increases the amount of oxygen in the blood. Delores Krieger, developer of Therapeutic Touch, ran three tests with healers and discovered that healing touch increased oxygen in hemoglobin by 12 percent (Krieger, *Therapeutic Touch*). These elevated oxygen levels may explain why praying for surgical patients produces such good surgical results.

Healing energy can be transmitted through electrical wire. A physician's wife wove electrical wiring through two vests that were connected together by wiring. Healer Olga Worrall wore one vest and an ill person whom Olga had never met down the hospital corridor wore the other. Physicians using instruments monitored a healing flow going through the wire. The ill woman became instantly well. (This was described by physicist John Zimmerman in an unpublished paper, 1988.)

The brain waves of a woman who was being prayed for without her knowledge showed significant changes. While a cooperating physician was recording a woman's brain waves, her prayer group prayed for her. The woman remained unaware of the prayers, but her recorded brain waves dramatically changed. In the process, the symptoms of the medical conditions for which she was seeing the doctor disappeared. Brain waves play an important part role in spiritual healing.

Healing energy is extremely stable. The qualities of the healing energy in healer-treated substances are different from those of any known energy source. The energy neither dissipates nor contaminates adjacent bottles of water. Healer-treated water and cotton cloth continue to emit the same level of healing energy two years later. This means that isolated healing energy is the most stable, storable known form of active energy. The energy of holy relics is also stable and storable.

Healing energy dissipates when imparted to living organisms. When healing energy is imparted to living organisms, it is rapidly used and diminishes in quantity. When Ambrose and Olga Worrall in Baltimore, Maryland, offered absent prayer for a blade of ryegrass in Atlanta, it rapidly accelerated growth for 11 hours to a maximum of 830 percent of normal. The growth enhancement then diminished for the next 36 hours, reaching a low of two times normal rate, where it remained for two weeks. (This was reported by Lee Poulas in *Miracles and Other Realities*, 1992.)

Healers prevent disease from occurring. In Bernard Grad's "Healing of Induced Goiters in Mice Experiment," mice were deprived of iodine and fed goitrogen thiouracil to induce goiters. Two healers treated the mice through touch-healing, preventing the goiters from occurring.

Mice rapidly used healing energy. Bernard Grad reports that the healing energy imparted to laboratory mice was so rapidly used that a healer had to hold the mice an hour at a time to maintain the necessary healing threshold of energy. Dr. Grad attributed this to the rapid metabolism of mice.

Prayers for healing of some persons can cause negative results. Gerald Sullivan injected malaria into mice and asked three volunteers to handle them for healing. One of the handlers, a scoffing nonbeliever in healing, was the focus of the experiment. This unbelieving volunteer produced statistically negative healing effects on the mice. It has been observed that one unbeliever in a prayer group can nullify the efforts of the group's prayers for healing.

Some electromagnetic frequencies may produce disease. Robert O. Becker and Gary Selden noted in *The Body Electric: Electromagnetism and the Foundation of Life* (Quill, 1985) that there had been, in the previous ten years, a 100 percent increase in lymphoma, a 97 percent increase in testicular cancer, a 31 percent increase in breast cancer, a 142 percent increase in kidney cancer, and a 63 percent increase in colon cancer. The authors linked exposure to man-made electromagnetic fields to the diseases of chronic fatigue syndrome, AIDS, autism, sudden infant death syndrome, Alzheimer's disease, Parkinson's disease, cancer, and mental diseases. People with these diseases should respond well to healing energy as it cancels the effects of the electromagnetic fields.

The power of group prayer is the square of the number of persons praying. Physicist William A. Tiller of Stanford University provides a scientific theory on the power of the energy emitted by a coherent group energy field as the square of the number of people involved. Two people praying together is four prayer power, ten people praying is 100 prayer power, 1,000 people praying is 1,000,000 prayer power. I have attended hundreds of healing services. I always feel an enormous quantity of healing energy permeating the service. It is some multiple of the people present. If one billion people prayed for the same thing, they could generate 1,000,000,000,000,000,000 units of healing energy, which might become a creative force to transform our whole planet, erasing pollution from the air and water.

In the 1989 Chouhan clinical studies at Jipmer Hospital in Pondicherry, India (published in the *International Journal of Obstetrics and Gynecology*), we proved many theories of the healing energy and healing. Using myself as the healer, we videotaped the changing energy fields of the subjects'/healees' fingertips as they were healed, using an advanced form of Kirlian photography. The conditions we worked in were ideal for healing. I was an imposing figure, an American, a Christian clergyman, a huge person by Indian standards (six foot, two inches tall and weighing 210 pounds). The healees spoke no English. The following are the clinical results that were videotaped:

A viral infection quickly healed. One morning, while we were calibrating our equipment, a young female laboratory assistant came to work with all the beginning symptoms of an acute head cold. Dr. Chouhan asked me to heal her, and I touched her on the forehead and nape of her neck. The videotape showed it took only two seconds for her baseline blue energy field with a white edge to be filled with healing energy, showing as a pure white energy field and remaining at that intensity. At 89 seconds, she complained of the heat she was feeling in her body. Not knowing her language, I did not understand the complaint and she broke from my healing grasp, screaming in utter pain. About an hour after our healing session, all symptoms of her cold were gone. Subjectively, I knew at 85 seconds of the healing encounter that she had been healed. At that time I can be heard on the videotape saying, "She has been healed." Healers have reported such subjective sensing that a healing has been complete, but this was the first time that it had been clinically proven to be accurate.

A woman with chronic back pain treated. The woman had traveled from more than a hundred miles away to see me. She had had constant spinal pain for ten years and her treatment had included two unsuccessful surgeries. I touched the nape of her neck and the base of her spine. Her baseline energy field was blue with a white halo. Later, watching the video, I saw that at three seconds of healing touch her energy field was transformed by the healing energy into a bright white. I had three sessions of ten minutes with her at 1 P.M. each day. She came the second and third day with her energy field showing up as bright white. The healing energy must have been there for the previous 24 hours. On the third day, in the midst of our healing encounter, she reported the complete alleviation of all symptoms. This was the first time in ten years she had been free of spinal pain. She glowed as she hugged me. My personal experience is that this type of healing consistently occurs with back conditions, trauma injuries, and presurgical healing preparations. Now I know that a person glows with a white human energy field when I apply touch-healing to them.

Precancerous test subject healed. Through fingertip bioelectrographic images, Dr. Chouhan had diagnosed precancerous cervical cancer in a young women he had tested. If left untreated, she would physically have cancer in three to six months. Here we used touch-healing as the primary treatment mode. As I touched her on the forehead and the nape of the neck, I subjectively sensed a resistance to the healing flow about eight minutes into the session. I can be heard on the videotape commenting, "She is not receiving the healing flow, but I will continue for a few more minutes." Just short of ten minutes, I commented, "She has begun receiving the healing flow."

It was a week later before I viewed the videotape. It showed nothing happening to her energy field until nine minutes and 45 seconds, when, like an explosion, the healing energy transformed her energy field into a bright white. I had been wrong in my interpretation. During the first nine minutes and 45 seconds, the healing energy had been entering her energy field and finally reached quantities that transformed it. Further fingertip bioelectrography showed that her energy field did not have the cancerous characteristics. She had been healed of her precancerous condition.

Summary of the Characteristics of Healing Energy

1. Healer-charged bottled water, wool, cotton, and gauze can be used for healing.

2. Healer-charged bottled water, wool, cotton, and gauze do not diminish their charge when stored for two years.

3. Naval physicists found frequencies that induced and healed cancer. A frequency generator used a 5.xxx hertz frequency to induce cancer in mice. Then it subjected the mice to the 8 hertz frequency and they got well.

4. Healing energy produces the optimum conditions for life.

5. Healing energy increases the amount of oxygen in the blood.

6. Healing energy can be transmitted through electrical wire.

7. The brain waves of a woman who was being prayed for without her knowledge showed significant changes.

8. Healing energy is extremely stable.

9. Healing energy dissipates when imparted to living organisms.

10. The high metabolism of mice rapidly uses up healing energy.

11. The prayers or healing touch of some persons can cause negative results.

12. Some electromagnetic frequencies may produce disease.

13. The power of group prayer is the square of the number of persons praying.

14. The healing of a cold took place in less than an hour.

15. The healing energy lasted for 24 hours with a woman with back pain.

16. Healing is not instant. It took 48 hours for the woman to be healed of back pain.

17. When a precancerous person was healed, it took nine minutes and 45 seconds to transform her energy field to the intense white of the healing energy.

18. At healing touch, in most cases, the normal human blue energy field changes in two to three seconds to a white energy field about twice the normal blue field's size.

19. Healing results are mainly due to the quality of the healing energy at 7.83 hertz, not the quantity.

20. If the average person provides two volts of healing energy, then two people praying produce four volts of healing energy—that's energy squared. So a thousand people praying produce four million volts of healing energy.

21. Loving concern and intention attune the healing energy.

My Own Experience in 30 Years of Practicing Healing

- If the body is healthy and does not need life energy, healing touch transfers no healing energy.

- The healing energy continues to be therapeutically present for about 48 hours. It is used up by the healing process and must be constantly replenished to a therapeutic quantity, just like a medication. An acutely ill person may need healing two or three times a day to maintain a therapeutic level of healing energy.

- You know the body is filled with a therapeutic level of healing energy when, after a few minutes, you take your hand away, shake it, and return it to position. If you feel no energy or heat at the site, no more healing flow is necessary.

- When a person senses intense heat or tingling during the healing encounter, a complete healing has usually taken place.

- When healing touch is applied to any part of the body, it travels to wherever it is needed.

- Emotional pain in body tissue hampers the usefulness of healing energy by changing the frequency to a nonhealing one. This stops any therapeutic effect.

This scientific picture helps us practice healing intelligently and confidently. This picture of healing is much different from what most people think.

Remember to use ERT before practicing healing. This is because emotional pain alters the frequency of the healing energy, making it not work.

European clinical reports of medical conditions responding well to touch-healing include: AIDS, allergies, anxiety, arthritic pain, asthma, bedwetting, benign tumors, brain bleeding, brain conditions, chronic illnesses, coronary insufficiency, deafness in children, disc displacement, ear infections, female disorders, gallbladder diseases, gastric conditions, ulcers, headaches, heart muscle damage, hypochondria, hysteria, nervous system disorders, nutritional disorders, obsessive-compulsive neurosis, ovarian disorders, ovarian cyst, prostate cancer, psychosomatic diseases, respiratory disorders, sinus infections, skin diseases, sterility, spinal root nerve irritation, stomach/intestinal problems, and stress disorders.

13

Bless the Children

Jenny reports: "I did ERT with a seven-year-old boy who had had several bad emotional experiences and had been acting out inappropriately with other children his age and younger. After two ERT sessions, the inappropriate behavior discontinued and he also quit blaming his mother for his father leaving him. His behavior changed dramatically at school, church, and home, and he was able to return to a public school environment. He began to catch up with his schoolwork and his reading level improved."

This chapter is aimed at motivating you to bless the children. You must learn to practice Emotional Release Therapy with children. After an ERT session, children glow with happiness. They tell you, "I have never felt so good in my life."

I joyously write this chapter! For three decades as a parish clergyman, I helplessly watched little children suffer emotionally. Counseling helped. Holding them helped. But their emotional pain was still there.

I remember being left alone with eight-year-old Johnny to tell him that his father had just died in a car accident.

I remember being alone with four young children whose mother had just died of cancer.

I remember comforting my crying five-year-old daughter, Claudia, in my arms after she had a traumatic experience at school.

I remember trying to comfort a severely depressed ten-year-old girl who had just flunked the fourth grade.

I remember helping 14-year-old Sean deal with his anger after the divorce of his parents.

I was troubled as I observed that most parents and professionals had fewer skills than I for helping emotionally hurting children. But, here and now, I feel enormous joy because every parent and teacher—any caring person—now has the potential to remove a child's emotional pain and traumas with ERT. Here are a few testimonials that illustrate this.

• Former ERT client and student Jim of Wadsworth, Ohio, tells this simple story with profound ramifications. He wrote: "After I practiced ERT on my 15-year-old daughter, her emotional balance quickly returned when she got upset. Her emotional upsets are not nearly as intense as they were."

• Jill of Oakwood Village, Ohio: "I came to my first ERT session with Dr. Weston feeling curious and left feeling peaceful and lighter. It improved my life by making me more peaceful. So, knowing how to do it, I began practicing ERT with my son. My son, John, was diagnosed with ADHD in 2003. I did ERT with him three nights in a row after learning it at Walter Weston's seminar. Following ERT, his behavior and attention improved to the point where he no longer needed his Daily Progress Report. This was after two summers of very expensive day camps for children with his disorder. My son has never been on ADHD medication, but he has had psychosocial intervention."

• Former student Jan Myers of Coshocton, Ohio, uses ERT with her whole family. "I use ERT on my six-year-old son, Max, whenever he appears to be getting frustrated or edgy—or if he is getting on my nerves, I know it is a good time for Emotional Release Therapy. It immediately calms him. We usually do ERT at bedtime after we say our prayers. I used ERT with my baby, Maggie, when she was teething. I also use it when she appears irritated. After ERT, she is so much better. Honestly, for mothers, I think this is a wonderful way to deal with parenting stress. ERT calms both mother and children. I also work with my husband periodically."

• Carol Adams of Lyndhurst, Ohio, reports on the physical healing of her son: "A few weeks ago, my 11-year-old son, Brian, was playing with friends, one of whom was throwing small, noisy firecrackers up against the side of a building. The firecrackers explode when they hit something hard and a piece of one flew into my son's eye, either lodging in his eye, scratching it, or burning it. His friend's mother rinsed Brian's eye and checked for dirt in and around the eye area. On our ride home, Brian cried almost continuously. At home, I decided to do ERT and physical healing. Just a few minutes after our session, the crying stopped and he became engrossed in watching TV. A while later he came to me saying that he felt no pain in his eye. He said it felt like nothing had happened to his eye at all. Thank God!"

• Rev. Jim of Warren, Ohio, practiced ERT on a six-year-old boy: "His mother brought him to me because he would cry every time she'd get in the car and go away, afraid that she'd get into a car accident and never come back. That was three weeks ago and he no longer cries like that."

Shortly after I discovered ERT, my granddaughter Melissa, then nine years old and diagnosed with ADD, was staying with us for the weekend. Though an intelligent child, Melissa was a borderline student who seldom did her homework. At home, she was uncooperative and sassy. That Friday evening, she sadly complained to me that she had never had a friend.

The next morning, she requested ERT. I sat beside her on the couch and in three minutes she had released all the emotional pain of her short life. Afterward, her face glowed with happiness as she exclaimed, "Grandpa, I feel wonderful! I have never felt this good in my life!"

Two weeks later, when I visited her home, she immediately jumped into my arms and excitedly whispered into my ear, "Grandpa, I have my first two friends upstairs in my bedroom. Come and meet them." I did. Then I went to the kitchen and talked to her mother. I asked, "How's Melissa doing?" She replied, "Dad, I don't know what happened, but

Melissa has completely changed. She's behaving well, just like her sisters. She's finally doing her homework and bringing home good grades."

A mother phoned for help for her 12-year-old daughter, Tiffany, who in the past year had been expelled from four different schools for behavioral problems. She was also failing most of her subjects.

Tiffany came to me with obvious reluctance. She was sulking as we began our ERT session. I encouraged her by saying, "You don't have to like me, but I promise that you are going to be feeling wonderfully happy in just a few minutes."

She released her emotional pain for almost half an hour. Afterward, she looked peaceful and happy. She shyly smiled, thanked me warmly, and left.

A few days later her mother phoned me, saying, "I can't believe it! Tiffany wants to see you again."

Tiffany greeted me with affection as we began our second ERT session. Afterward, glowing with happiness, she hugged me and kissed me on the cheek.

A few weeks later, Tiffany's mother reported, "It's a miracle, Dr. Weston. Tiffany is behaving well, just like my other children. For the first time, she loves going to school and is getting good grades. We are talking to each other all the time. I have watched what you are doing with her and can't believe such a simple thing can do what it is doing. Thank you!"

Since then I have practiced Emotional Release Therapy with dozens of children. Every one of them has been completely transformed.

An infant with colic and diaper rash, who cried all the time and slept at irregular intervals, was immediately freed of these symptoms.

A five-year-old who wet the bed took one session of ERT to stop.

After ERT, a 15-year-old boy who was filled with anger and had been physically violent in both school and home no longer was angry or violent.

After ERT, the academic performance and behavior of numerous children and youth dramatically improved.

The implications are clear. A child's unacceptable grades and behavior are primarily due to emotional pain and destructive emotional states. Their emotional pain keeps students from achieving up to potential by affecting brain function, so they are unable to remember their school lessons or focus on studying.

Emotional pain appears to be a primary cause for unacceptable behavior, because it destroys behavioral judgment and controls. Removing emotional pain results in better grades and more acceptable behavior.

Emotional Release Therapy addresses the enormous issues of why Johnny can't learn and can't behave appropriately. Any parent, grandparent, sibling, teacher, or student can learn to practice ERT with children.

Recently, a 35-year-old woman came to me because she had daily been haunted by an event that had occurred 30 years before, when she was five years old. She had been riding her bike at a large family reunion when she fell off and hurt herself. Everyone laughed! Now, most of us wouldn't be wounded for 30 years by such an event, but Mary was. I worked with her for ten minutes and her haunting was over and she was at peace. We worked further and she released emotional pain from throughout her life.

Many people live with their emotional trauma for years, not knowing how to get rid of it.

ERT can help children in a number of ways:

• Failing children can learn up to potential after ERT.

• Disorderly children live responsibly after ERT.

• Using ERT on juvenile delinquents can end their errant behavior.

• Using ERT and ERT BodyTalk with infants up to six months old can heal children of birth defects.

• Using ERT and ERT BodyTalk with infants up to six months old can possibly remove the emotional trauma from the womb and early life to increase their intelligence.

It is truly a gift of love. Why not practice ERT with children?

14

With Whom to Practice ERT

Professionals who already work with people have no problem finding clients with whom to practice ERT. Such professionals include people in the medical field, psychotherapists, social workers, schoolteachers, clergy, and healers. For all these professionals, ERT restores people to health and wholeness. For healers, it answers the age-old question of why some people are not healed. The answer is that people who are filled with emotional pain do not respond well to healing efforts. Remove a person's emotional pain and almost everyone is healed.

You Must Practice ERT within a Week of Finishing This Book

I conclude workshops by telling my students that they must practice Emotional Release Therapy with at least two people in the coming week. Why? Because if they don't, they will probably never practice ERT. The same challenge faces people who have read this book. If you do not work with at least two people within a week of completing this book, you are not likely ever to practice ERT with others. It takes confidence and boldness to practice ERT. If you lack these, use ERT on yourself to remove these barriers. Then let your new self practice ERT.

If You Are Not a Professional

There are many people to approach with the purpose of practicing ERT. First are family members. Practice it on children in the family. Promise them that they will feel wonderful after ERT. Practice it with friends and coworkers. Practice with grieving people at least a month after the death of a loved one. Practice it with hospitalized people. If you know of people who are taking medications for depression or anxiety, begin by telling them you have learned a new technique that might help them. Everyone possesses emotional pain so everyone needs Emotional Release Therapy. If you are in a community group or church, you might offer to teach a group to practice ERT.

Part IV

Special Techniques

15

ERT with Infants and Children

Working with infants is so rewarding and so easy. When infants behave poorly, it is because they are hurting.

Some 25 years ago, I baptized a six-month-old baby. Several months later, the mother of the baby attended the mother's support group that I led. She stayed afterward and talked to me privately. She said, "My second son was not like my first son. My first son was perfect, but my second son had colic and diaper rash. He slept through the day and kept me awake at night. He screamed and cried for no reason at all. At times, I got so upset with him that I wanted to throw him against the wall and kill him. But then you baptized him when he was six months old and he immediately stopped all of his destructive behavior and became a model child, just like his older brother. Thank you."

I know I am a healer. I know the Sacraments have great spiritual power. But I was shocked by this healing. It meant, first, that children can be born with qualities that produce disruptive behavior and illness. Perhaps during pregnancy a child is physically and/or emotionally traumatized. Second, it is easy to return a child to health and wholeness through ERT and ERT BodyTalk.

Ralph DeOrio, the first Roman Catholic priest to become a faith healer in the twentieth century, healed a six-month-old mentally retarded child, causing his facial features and brain to become that of a normal child. Later, in elementary school, the boy was discovered to be a gifted child. The healing occurred during two sessions. Father DeOrio held him in a healing mass in Massachusetts and a few weeks later came to his home in Chicago, where he had another healing mass in the parent's home.

An infant, Bill, was born with physical deformities. I practiced ERT and ERT BodyTalk three times with him when he was one week old. I also charged healing towels and healing water, which his mother used. Within a month, all the birth deformities were gone.

Debra, 14 months old, had diaper rash and allergies. She slept days and was awake nights. She cried often without any apparent reason and was plainly unhappy. Following one session of Emotional Release Therapy, all symptoms of poor behavior ended and she became a happy child.

Shari, nine, was failing in school and her behavior was poor. After one ERT session her grades improved and she behaved well.

Jerry, six, was the fourth member of the same family I had worked with. First I worked with his mother and then with his two teenage siblings, practicing ERT with them. At that time, he was the youngest child with whom I had ever practiced ERT.

He sat on my lap with his mother looking on. I said, "Do you have emotional pain to heal?"

He said, "Yes, a boy at school keeps beating me up. I'm afraid of him and I'm angry."

I said, "Let me put my hand on your heart and you can give your hurt to me any way you can."

Jerry closed his eyes, took a deep breath, and exhaled strongly. I felt the heat of his release enter my hand. He then took another deep breath and exhaled. He said, "I feel great, Mister. I released my anger and then I released my fear. I feel fine. Thanks, Mister." And he jumped from my lap and ran to his mother.

Infants, toddlers, elementary school children, and youth respond well to Emotional Release Therapy. They are a joy to work with and the results are spectacular.

With infants, the mother either holds them or they are in a crib. I place my flattened hand on their heart. I say, "Release your emotional pain into my hand on your heart." I always feel the heat of their release. Then I use a prayer blessing. With my hand on their heart, I pray something like, "Be filled with God's peace and love." Afterward, they often smile or laugh.

The first time I did it, I felt the heat of the infant's release. I said to myself, infants understand what I am saying on some level. I have worked with infants from the moment of birth.

Remember, newborns with physical and mental handicaps or problems can be restored to full health with ERT up to six months old.

I have used ERT BodyTalk with them. After ERT, I place my hand on top of their head and pray, "May healing flow from my hand, entering your head and healing your brain, flowing into your torso and making it whole, down your arms and making them whole, down your legs and making them whole. Restore every cell in your body and make them whole and healthy. Thank you. Amen."

Elementary age children respond well to regular ERT and ERT BodyTalk. All of them comment about feeling good, wonderful, and at peace. If they don't respond well to regular ERT, I ask them to respond any way they can.

I practiced ERT on my grandchildren. I did it with nine-year-old Megan and 11-year-old Jessica. When I finished with them, their four-year-old brother, Matthew, ran up to me, holding his hand over his heart, and said, "Hurts."

My granddaughter Jessica said, "Let me do Matthew, Grandpa." She modeled herself after me and did ERT with Matthew.

She placed her hand on his chest and said, "Matthew, choose a color and place it in your heart. Now release the feeling of your hurts into my hand on your heart." Matthew released for about five minutes and said he was done. Jessica then said, "Now release your anger toward family members." He released for another five minutes. Jessica then said, "Be filled with God's peace and love." Afterward, Matthew just smiled.

If an 11-year-old can practice ERT after watching it done with her sister and herself, surely all you readers can bring joy to infants, toddlers, elementary children, and youth.

Remember, children release much faster than adults. They also have shorter histories of emotional pain to release.

16

ERT without Touching

Some professionals are not permitted to touch people. Psychologists are not permitted to touch clients. Schoolteachers have to be cautious about touching people. Some men and women do not like to be touched, especially in the chest area. You do not have to touch people to practice ERT. You as the ERT practitioner can sit behind a desk if you so choose. You can work with a client sitting in a chair ten feet away.

How to Do ERT without Touching

The ERT practitioner and the client sit in separate chairs, not touching each other. You as the ERT practitioner place your dominant hand on your own heart. The client is asked to put her dominant hand over her own heart.

You say, "Let us pray. God help _____ [client's name] release her emotional pain into her hand and then let me receive the emotional pain into my hand. Thank you. Amen."

You then say, "Let's close our eyes. Now, I want you to choose a color and place it in your heart. Now, release the feelings of your emotional pain into the color in your heart. I am going to receive your released emotional pain into my hand from your hand." This is the only difference between touch and nontouch ERT.

You go on to say, "Now, release your emotional pain into your heart. That's it. I can feel release of the heat of your toxic emotions entering my hand. Keep releasing your emotional pain into your hand and I will receive them into my hand." Rinse your hand when it grows hot.

You can practice ERT or ERT BodyTalk in that way. Your hand feels the release from the client's hand. You rinse your hand periodically in salt-water to dissolve the toxic emotions collected in it.

You can do the prayer blessing at the end by sending it from your heart into your client's heart, praying, "God, fill _____ [client's name] with your peace and love. Thank you. Amen."

When you begin, you'll often do a double take as you feel the heat of her release coming into your hand. I am not speculating on why this occurs. I am just happy it does.

For ERT BodyTalk, place your hand on top of your head and ask your client to place her dominant hand on top of her head. Your healing hand keeps sending the healing energy into the client's hand and it will flow to wherever you direct it in the client's body.

17

ERT over the Phone

I do most of my ERT over the phone without touching people. I am an author and a workshop leader, so people call me from all over for healing.

My first request for healing over the phone came from Arizona. A talk show host who interviewed me wanted me to do ERT with his wife. So I called her. She told me she was a massage therapist and a Reiki master. I thought, "Boy, is this ever going to be easy."

She called at our agreed time and was lying on her massage table as I had requested. I asked her to place her dominant hand on her heart. I told her my hand was on my heart.

Visualize a color. I said, "Visualize a color and place it in your heart. Now, release the feelings of your emotional pain into your heart and into your hand. I will receive the toxic emotions from your hand into my hand. Now, release your painful emotions into your heart and into your hand."

I immediately felt the release of heat into my hand. I thought, "It's working!" And we continued with ERT. It was easy!

Rinse your hand. I rinsed my hand in the saltwater bowl periodically to wash away the toxic emotions she was releasing.

Prayer blessing. I gave her the prayer blessing at the end. "Fill _____ [client's name] with peace and love. Amen." I had not discovered ERT BodyTalk yet, so I did not do it.

It would be good to have a headset for your phone so you don't tire your arm holding the receiver to your ear.

If I had done ERT BodyTalk, I would have continued with my hand on my heart and said, "Leave your hand on your heart. We'll go through your body. We are going to cleanse every cell in your body. Close your eyes. Place your dominant hand on your heart."

Talk to the body one organ/part at a time. Say, "Brain, release your emotional pain, your physical discomfort, and your dysfunction into my hand when I count to one. 3, 2, 1, release."

The release is delayed compared to ERT. If the release is strong, repeat the procedure.

Do this with the brain, ears, eyes, sinuses, nose, throat, lungs, heart, liver, pancreas, spleen, esophagus, stomach, intestines, bladder, kidneys, reproductive organs, sexual organs, nerves, muscles, bone joints, blood vessels, blood, skin, and so forth. Rinse your hand in saltwater often.

Say, "Release your emotional pain, your physical discomfort, and your dysfunction into my hand when I count to one. 3, 2, 1, release."

Filling Your Body with God's Healing Power

Hand position. Close your eyes. Place your dominant hand on top of your head. Your hand will become less tired if you are lying down.

Pray. "God, may your healing power flow from my hand into her brain. Thank you. Amen."

Talk to the brain. Say to the brain, "Brain, open a door and let this healing flow in." Mentally visualize it flowing into her.

Talk to God. "God's healing power, flow throughout her brain, restoring all brain functions and filling them with your peace. Amen." Imagine it flowing throughout her brain.

Do the same thing with the body's organs/parts. Do this for the eyes, ears, sinuses, nose, mouth, throat, lungs, heart, liver, gallbladder, pancreas, spleen, esophagus, stomach, intestines, bladder, kidneys, reproductive organs, sexual organs, nerves, muscles, bone joints, blood vessels, blood, skin, and so on.

With your dominant hand on top of your head, pray: "God, may your healing power flow from my hand into her _____ [body part], flow throughout her ____ [body part], restoring her health, and filling it with your peace. Amen." Imagine it flowing throughout her _____ [body part].

Healing Body Sections

Place your hand on top of your head and pray: "God, may your healing power flow from my hand into her brain, renewing every cell in her head, flow down her right arm into her fingers, renewing every cell in her right arm, may it flow down her left arm into her fingers, renewing every cell in her left arm, may it flow from her brain down her throat into the whole torso, renewing every cell in her torso, may it flow down her right leg to her toes, renewing every cell in her right leg, may it flow down her left leg to her toes, renewing every cell in her left leg. Amen."

18

ERT with Pets and Other Animals

I have not worked with many animals, but I have found that animals are easier to heal than humans. Twenty years ago, I healed my first animal, a pet cat. It was in a remote rural area. The owner only said the cat hadn't moved in three days. Then she left me alone with an almost dead cat. I placed my hand on the cat's head and prayed for its healing, leaving my hand there for five minutes. I did not see the owner before leaving. The next morning she phoned and said the cat was back to normal, eating and exploring the house.

Horses

I was working with a depressed woman who told me her horse would have to be destroyed because it had a painful incurable hoof disease in all four hoofs. I agreed to try curing it. We went out to the stable and she tied the horse between two posts on both sides so the horse couldn't move. I then worked on the hoofs. I put my healing hand about one-quarter inch from each hoof and took away its pain. Then I did healing touch directly on each hoof. In all, it took about 15 minutes. A week later, the woman phoned me to say that the veterinarian had examined the hoofs and had been amazed that the horse was well.

A wealthy man in Michigan asked me to work with six racing colts before my workshop in Lansing. They were too wild to be trained and were going to be destroyed. We drove two hours to the stable, where I attempted to practice ERT with each. I had to ask where a horse's heart is. On each horse, I placed my healing hand on the heart and asked the horse to release its emotional pain. The horses each responded by releasing a lot of heat from the heart. I concluded with a prayer blessing offering the horse God's peace and love. They seemed to be telepathic. The horses' lives were spared.

Dogs and Cats

In doing ERT with dogs and cats, I have given directions similar to those I give to humans, without mentioning the color focus, however. Each animal released its emotional pain; each accepted the healing flow.

Several had cancer. One had a birth defect. Several had injuries. What struck me is that the owners told me their pets were grouchy and would likely resist my touch. But just the opposite happened. They accepted my first touch with hearty warmth, somehow knowing that I was going to help them. Some were emotionally wounded, acting strangely or being very quiet and alone. But they were emotionally healed.

I remember one dog with deep affection. He was a German shepherd. The owner warned me that the dog bit anyone who touched him. He had a birth defect. Both his hind legs were wasting away. He dragged himself with his front legs. He was nine months old. I looked into his eyes with compassion and touched him in the heart area. He grinned back at me. I did Emotional Release Therapy on him and he became limp. I then touched his legs for touch-healing, praying for his health.

The owner and the dog left my home. Two weeks later, the owner phoned. All four legs worked normally and dog and owner were taking long walks in the park.

Dogs Are Healers

Dogs are healers, too. They emit the 7.83 hertz healing frequency to their loved ones who are hurting. A researcher measured a dog's energy emissions and discovered their healing capabilities.

How to Heal Animals

I touch them on the heart, which is between their front legs. I ask them to release their emotional pain into my hand. They do. Then I do touch-healing prayer on the part of the body that is ill. I've worked with about two dozen animals. All have been healed. Let's go through the process.

Place your hand on the animal's heart. Pray aloud: "God, help _____ [animal's name] release its emotional pain into my hand. Amen."

Then say to the dog almost the same thing you would say to humans, "Release your emotional and physical pain into my hand that you might be well." And they do. (Are they telepathic?) Rinse your hand in saltwater.

Then bless them, "God, fill this animal with your peace and love. Amen."

19

Filling People with Positive Personal Traits

Write down the personal traits with which you wish to be filled—things such as love, peace, happiness, or fairness. Practice ERT and prayer blessings on yourself with the personal traits you desire. Repeat this day after day until you feel results and know it works for you. You should feel these personal traits becoming a part of you.

Surround yourself with that which will help to transform you.

1. Pray daily for the personal traits you desire.

2. Make sure your family has had ERT and is happy.

3. Make sure your job is life-giving. If it is filled with anger, hostility, suspicion, or doubts about your abilities, change the atmosphere by practicing ERT with people who can change the place into one with good vibes.

4. Take part in activities that permeate you with the personal traits you desire.

5. Listen to classical music and easy listening music. Avoid rock music because it can cause anxiety.

6. Read books that inspire you.

7. Do not watch violent movies, television shows, or plays.

8. Do not play destructive video games.

9. Do not associate with people who do not have the personal traits you desire. We become like the company we keep as their destructive energy fields permeate us.

10. Join churches and community groups with people who have the personal traits you desire. You may at first feel uncomfortable with these people if you lack the personal traits they have, but hang in there.

If you try these, let me know how things turn out.

Or you can have someone practice Emotional Release Therapy with you and close with a prayer blessing, filled with the traits you desire. Provide the ERT therapist with the list of your desired traits so she can bless you with them. After the prayer blessing, sit for a minute or two with the ERT therapist's hand on your breastbone. See if it makes a difference.

Part V

Experiencing Empathy and God

20

Closed Hearts Lack Empathy

Then she said to him, "How can you say, 'I love you,' when your heart is not with me?"

—Judg. 16:15

I have no feelings. My heart is empty.

—An ERT client

Getting in touch with your emotions is one of the first steps in personal growth and maturity. Closed hearts do not feel emotions. They lack empathy and compassion. The closed heart is a thinking-only heart. It is not balanced by emotions. It rarely feels emotions.

The heart is the primary location where emotions are felt. A heart that is emotionally impaired or closed is incapable of fully feeling its own emotions or the emotions of others.

When, prior to an ERT session, a person states that he feels nothing and his heart is empty, I arrive at one of three possible conclusions.

First, the person is depressed, grief-stricken, or in emotional shock. These emotional states block one's awareness of emotions. Fortunately, during Emotional Release Therapy these emotions can be released and the heart can again feel emotions. These new-felt emotions can be released during the same ERT session.

Second, the person is suffering from so many emotional traumas that he has protectively closed his heart in order to survive. After being assured that it is now safe to feel emotional traumas one last time—because after they are released they will be gone forever—he is always able to do so. Sometimes talking about the events of his emotional history must precede this. He may also need to talk about his emotional history during ERT.

Third, the person may be on a medication or a recreational drug that deadens the emotions. If it is a medication, he is still able to release, but the release feels dulled as it enters the practitioner's hand. If a recreational drug impedes release, I tell the person to come back later at a drug-free time.

With these conditions, emotional release produces a healthy emotional heart. The emotionally healthy heart is able to give and to receive love, to feel the pain of self and others, to respond compassionately to the emotional pain of others, and to interact emotionally with people in all relationships.

Finally, a thinking-type personality finds it difficult to feel emotions. He mostly operates in the thinking mode. This usually begins in childhood and accelerates through the years to the place where he is all but devoid of emotional awareness. In effect, he has closed his heart to feeling emotional information in self and others. He can still receive and feel the love, affection, and support of others but is unable to reciprocate by giving others his love, affection, and support. He is unable to understand the yearning of his loved ones to interact on an emotional basis. This may leave him feeling frustrated and unappreciated.

The problem is that he can't interact emotionally because the closed heart lacks the ability to emotionally feel. His strongest emotional responses are likely to be anger and annoyance. Because he has rarely felt them, he does not value the emotions of self or others.

This profile can fit men or women. If one marital partner is a feeling type and the other a thinking type, this is bound to be a major contributing factor to an unhappy marriage and divorce.

Males do have some fixed emotions. There is grumpiness! There is anger! Almost every male has a huge reservoir of anger within him that he can tap into at any time. Talk about this in a room full of women and they will howl in glee at the acknowledgment of it.

Some men are a bit ashamed of their anger, embarrassed that they blow up at the women in their lives. Well, men, you don't have to put up with it any longer. You don't have to be ashamed again. You can drain this huge reservoir of anger during Emotional Release Therapy and seldom be angry again.

Can thinking-type people change and learn to use their hearts to love? Yes. But first they must recognize their need to do so. They must see that the reward for doing so is well worth the effort. Here are four suggested motivations:

1. Using the heart to love enhances immensely the joy and satisfaction of family life.

2. Using the heart to love enhances workplace situations that value sensitive people.

3. Using the heart to love makes one immensely happy.

4. Using the heart to love makes one healthier and live longer.

Should a thinking-type person recognize the need to be more emotionally aware, there is now a solution using ERT. This involves three steps.

The first step is experiencing Emotional Release Therapy. After releasing their emotional pain, thinking-type people must be guided into releasing all their anger and negative self-images. Second, during that same session, they need to practice opening their heart to sense the feelings of others. This gives them the skill of having control over their heart, which they can open and close at will.

Finally, they need to be coached by a loved one who will help them practice opening their heart in love in various real-life situations. These situations include with their coach, in various gatherings of loved ones and friends, and in some chosen situation of nurturing or caring for someone.

This process also includes being taught simple listening and nurturing skills.

Eric and Rachel came to me for marital counseling. My approach began with ERT with each of them to remove their emotional pain and bad feelings toward each other. Listening to the issues that troubled their marriage followed.

The main issue was Rachel's disillusionment over Eric not being more affectionate and caring. They both agreed to the preceding approach with ERT and successfully followed it through. Eric attained an emotionally healthy heart.

Men, why not give it a try? Afterward, your mother, wife, and daughter(s) will love and cherish you far more than they do now.

First, people with the thinking heart, the closed heart, must have basic Emotional Release Therapy, either with someone else conducting it or doing it themselves. The very act of experiencing ERT will put them in an emotional mood.

Second, they must release all anger toward family, friends, work situations, and themselves.

Third, they must discuss emotional relationships with family members. It is useful to have a woman's help with this.

Fourth, they have to learn to care for someone, coached by the ERT practitioner.

Fifth, they should be taught by a female ERT practitioner simple listening and nurturing skills.

21

Closed Hearts Cannot Experience God

When you search for me, you will find me; if you seek me with all your heart.

—Jer. 29:13

Oh, is that what God feels like? I have always wondered about that. Boy, that felt good!

—A 35-year-old man whose face glowed with spiritual bliss after experiencing God for the first time during Emotional Release Therapy

I visited with Candy, a depressed pastor, who was in a psychiatric ward. She began to weep uncontrollably. Through her tears, Candy moaned, "Not only am I depressed, it is like God has deserted me. For the first time in my life, God isn't there." Other depressed people I've encountered have said that God isn't there for them, as have people in grief.

While I was visiting Millie, a recently widowed woman, she bitterly complained through tears, "Not only have I lost my husband, God isn't here with me either. God has always daily been with me as I prayed. Now, he is gone, too." I have heard similar complaints from dozens of widows.

What do depression and grief have in common? An impaired heart. It is through a healthy heart that we experience God.

I wondered why women came to Bible study and spiritual growth groups, when maybe only ten percent of participants were men. Why do women have such an interest in experiencing God when most men don't? Vividly impressed in my mind are scenes of women in the church casually standing in a circle and glowing with happiness as they shared their experiences of God among themselves.

At the same time, I observe their husbands standing apart from them, bored and shuffling their feet because they seemingly could not relate to any of the words the women were speaking. It is always obvious to me that these men have never experienced God.

During a counseling appointment, Kevin, a 35-year-old schoolteacher, shared the following: "Pastor, I come to church to be supportive of my wife and children and because of the loving fellowship, but I have never experienced God. Can you help me experience God?"

At that time, I had no clue how to help. But Emotional Release Therapy has now taught me that he must have had a closed heart that was incapable of experiencing God.

I have never forgotten my childhood experience of hearing my pastor say during a sermon, "If only you will open your heart, you will know God!" I immediately identified with that. As a ten-year-old child, I had opened my heart and had been filled with God's spiritual bliss. As I recalled my pastor speaking those words, tears of joy once more streamed down my cheeks.

I had practiced ERT with 35-year-old Jack, giving him a prayer blessing, when Jack said he'd had a strange experience. He described the experience.

I chuckled, recognizing the strange experience, and said, "You've just experienced God."

Jack replied, "Oh, I've always wondered what God felt like. That felt good!"

I asked, "Would you like to experience God more fully?"

Jack answered, "Yes, I would."

With my hand on his heart, we resumed Emotional Release Therapy. I stated, "Put yourself in a relaxed state." I felt his relaxed state with my hand on his heart. I said, "I am filled with God and I am going to send you God." I sent him God.

He said, "That feels wonderful!"

"Now I am going to merge with you and God." I did.

We merged with God and each other. We shared spiritual bliss for 20 minutes, something I experience with about ten percent of my clients during ERT. Then it was over.

I explained how he could open his heart to God. Do ERT during a prayer service, while reading the Bible, while listening to sacred music, and in other places where you might experience God.

Through the years Jack and I have kept in contact with each other. He remains close to God.

I have never heard anyone talk about the fact that most men have never experienced God. Wives and mothers comment that the men in their lives are bored with the church and indifferent toward God.

No wonder! How would you like to sit through a church service designed specifically to help people experience God and never experience anything sacred through the music, the prayers, the rituals, the sermon?

Most men at an early age close their heart to God by choosing to be rational and logical. Or perhaps the male is affected by the male sex hormone testosterone into being rational rather than emotional. They don't value emotions. As children, they were chided by their fathers and others with the statement "Big boys don't cry!" They turned off their ability to feel emotions. They closed their hearts. People with closed hearts are incapable of experiencing God. How many people in our nation have never experienced God? Maybe 75 percent of all men have not experienced God. Plus millions of emotionally wounded women.

But now we have a new means for helping curious thinking-type people experience God for the first time. Emotional Release Therapy itself often includes the presence of God. This means opening your heart during ERT and being surprised by God in the process.

God may also be present as the ERT practitioner and client both open their hearts, causing their hearts to merge. The merging of any two or more hearts may produce powerful experiences of God. Like Jesus said, "Where two or more are gathered in my name, there am I in the midst of them."

I had this happen with my brother, Bernie. Our love for each other was extremely strong. But, other than that, we lived completely different lifestyles. I lived in Ohio; he lived in San Diego. From childhood, I loved God. From childhood, Bernie was angry with God. I was steadily experiencing God while Bernie never had and thus could not believe in God.

In 1987, when Bernie was dying of pancreatic cancer, he came from San Diego to live with my wife and me. When he came to me, he agreed to pray with me every morning and evening. This became important to him.

Three weeks later, three days before his death, Bernie experienced God for the first time. It was in the evening. We were in his darkened bedroom, he in his wheelchair and I sitting in front of him as we joined hands for our evening prayer.

It was a splendid experience! Early into the prayer, I felt the most beautiful love I had ever known. Sweet and gentle and deep. God was powerfully within me and the white mystic light filled my mind.

I heard my brother sobbing deeply as if from afar. And then I realized that I, too, was sobbing. After our prayer, the Holy Presence, the Sweet Love, and the Holy Light continued, seeming to go on endlessly. And then it was over.

We had shared identical experiences. Our hearts had been merged. Then Bernie uttered his first words of faith. In awe, he whispered, "If this is what it is like with God on the other side, I am no longer afraid to die. I will die in peace."

Two hearts merged more easily experience God.

If you wish to open your heart to God, here are some suggestions.

First, personally experience Emotional Release Therapy by doing Self-ERT. This alone may open your heart to God. If it doesn't, go to an ERT practitioner and experience ERT.

Second, go to a religious service and practice ERT in the midst of various religious rituals. You will be aware of God's presence this way.

Third, during private prayer or meditation or religious songs, practice ERT on yourself.

This concludes how to open your heart to God.

Part VI

Spirituality

22

Opposition to Emotional Release Therapy

I speculate that there have been a few cures for cancer that have never reached the public. After all, treating cancer is a multibillion-dollar-a-year industry. Think of all the people who would lose their jobs if there were no cancer patients. How do you destroy an innovative new invention that threatens the status quo? By shunning the inventor.

Two years ago, I was invited to speak about Emotional Release Therapy to a holistic health group at a hospital that is in the top 50 in the nation in treating many medical conditions. About 70 attentive listeners—doctors, nurses, administrators—gathered in the lecture room late one afternoon. As I finished my lecture on ERT, they gave me a standing ovation.

I was excited. Two department heads approached me afterward and said they would like to use ERT in their departments. I gave them my calling card with my e-mail address on it.

Sounds great, doesn't it? But the next day, I received e-mails from both department heads. They each said the same thing: "I have been forbidden to use Emotional Release Therapy in my department." Shunned!

The head psychologist in charge of psychotherapy for female veterans at a veterans hospital attended one of my weekend workshops. At the end of the workshop, Dr. Johnson gushed to me about Emotional Release Therapy.

A few days later, I phoned her at her office. "How's ERT doing with your veterans? Have you tried it yet with post-traumatic stress disorder?"

Dr. Johnson coolly replied, "I can't use it with my veterans. It is not among the treatments approved by the American Psychological Association." Then she gave me a bone to gnaw on. She said. "I have a woman veteran who has not responded well to treatment after a year's therapy. How would you like to work with her? Her name is Gloria."

Gloria came to my home for our session. She was warm, friendly, and very pretty. She explained that while in the army she had been raped by a whole array of men who were her superiors. She was struggling with post-traumatic stress disorder. Because of it, she couldn't work and was a very poor mother to her two children. Her husband was ready to divorce her.

Within minutes of her arrival, we were practicing Emotional Release Therapy. I could feel the warmth of her release of emotional pain enter my hand. She released steadily for 40 minutes before announcing, "I am done. I feel wonderful!"

"Gloria, I don't know if we got rid of all your emotional pain. So, if in the coming days, you again feel emotional pain, call me and we'll have another session together."

A few days later, she phoned me. She said, "I am completely back to my normal self. The emotional pain of the rapes is completely past. I don't even think about them now. My children and husband welcomed the new old me. I am resuming my career as an entertainer in two weeks by singing in your city at Sam's Place and I'd like you and your wife to come and hear me."

We did. My wife and I discovered that Gloria was a fabulous entertainer.

I called Dr. Johnson at the VA Hospital and reported my results. She said, "That's good," and hung up. In response to several subsequent calls from me, her secretary said she was not available.

I've been shunned by the Pentagon, rape crisis centers, battered women's shelters, the Red Cross, a hospice, school guidance counselors, psychologists, and medical doctors. I am telling you so you know that

Emotional Release Therapy is an innovative discovery that faces challenges to its acceptance. Institutions and professions cannot begin to understand what ERT does. Those who do understand don't want to change how services are delivered by hospitals, schools, social agencies, and doctor's offices. It will cost many professional workers their jobs, as ERT does things more easily and efficiently than they do it.

You may be in a position to enable ERT to be used in a professional setting. It will take ingenuity and courage to get ERT accepted. If you are in a position to do so, please enable Emotional Release Therapy. As it helped you, so can it help others.

All six billion people on this planet can use ERT. In war-ridden Bosnia or Afghanistan or Iraq, ERT could remove the wounds of war for whole nations. ERT needs to be accepted.

23

ERT in a Biblical Context

The good person out of the good treasure of the heart produces good, and the evil person out of evil treasure produces evil; for it is out of the abundance of the heart that the mouth speaks.

—Luke 6:45

They are darkened in their understanding, alienated from the life of God because of their ignorance and hardness of heart.

—Eph. 4:18

Now that you have purified your souls by your obedience to the truth so that you have genuine mutual love, love one another deeply from the heart.

—1 Pet. 1:22

I remain grounded in Christian faith, so my approach to Emotional Release Therapy comes from my own religious experiences and belief system. But my clients and students would never know this from what they experience during my ERT sessions or seminars.

Emotional Release Therapy is a technique or a process. It is religiously neutral. It can be used in any religious context. In my seminars, I have trained Christians, Jews, Muslims, Hindus, New Agers, and agnostics.

But anyone who undergoes or practices Emotional Release Therapy learns that it is almost always a spiritual experience. The content of the spiritual experience is similar for everyone, regardless of his or her faith tradition.

Biblical scholars agree that the word "heart" in the Bible is not referring literally to the heart but to the total spiritual essence of a person. Emotional Release Therapy agrees with this interpretation.

According to the ERT experience, when we open our hearts to God, God literally fills or dwells within the energy or location of the heart. When the heart has been emotionally traumatized or is closed, we cannot experience God's presence. If God is not present in the heart, goodness can still dwell there.

But, with the absence of God, when a person does evil deeds, his heart may become filled with evil, which is a dark energy that can deeply influence one's morality, thoughts, and actions. The presence of God in the heart protects a person from the dark energies' influence.

The heart molds a person's character. As Jesus states, "The good person out of the good treasure of the heart produces good, and the evil person out of evil treasure produces evil; for it is out of the abundance of the heart that the mouth speaks" (Luke 6:45).

The apostle Paul agreed with Jesus that the heart molds character, writing, "They are darkened in their understanding, alienated from the life of God because of their ignorance and hardness of heart" (Eph. 4:18).

The disciple Peter discerned that sacred love flows from the heart. "Now that you have purified your souls by your obedience to the truth so that you have genuine mutual love, love one another deeply from the heart" (1 Pet. 1:22).

The heart is the actual place where we experience God. As the prophet Jeremiah said of the Lord God, "When you search for me, you will find me; if you seek me with all your heart" (Jer. 29:13).

The psalmist prayed with this understanding, saying, "Create in me a clean heart, O God, and put a new and right spirit within me" (Ps. 51:10).

When Jesus said, "Blessed are the pure in heart, for they will see God" (Matt. 5:8), he knew something that I only learned through Emotional Release Therapy.

When during ERT a person releases his emotional pain and his fear, anger, and guilt, the heart becomes pure and open to "see God." What a marvelous transformative tool for salvation!

The heart is where we hold our commitment to God and take action based on faith. As Jesus quoted, "Out of the believer's heart shall flow rivers of living water" (John 7:38).

The heart is the basis for divinely knowing humans. "But the Lord said to Samuel, 'Do not look on his appearance or on the height of his stature, because I have rejected him; for the Lord does not see as mortals see; they look on the outward appearance, but the Lord looks on the heart'" (1 Sam. 16:7).

The apostle Paul wrote, "Indeed, the word of God is living and active, sharper than any two-edged sword, piercing until it divides soul from spirit, joints from marrow; it is able to judge the thoughts and intentions of the heart" (Heb. 4:12).

Forgiveness takes on new meaning with ERT. With ERT, you are able to release negative feelings toward others. Then forgiveness is easy because with ERT you release ill feelings toward those who have hurt you and no longer feel those feelings.

Salvation takes on new meaning, too. ERT opens your heart to God. It is no longer a struggle to find God. You just open your new heart to God.

ERT should precede baptism, confirmation, and weddings in the Christian traditions. It clears the negative and brings people closer to God.

I agree that when the Bible refers to the heart, it is referring to the essence of a person. The heart is where we experience God. Yet the heart, like a hologram, places the divine essence into every cell of the body.

The sacredness of the heart is also written as information in the human spiritual body. It resides in the fourth human energy field (one of seven) of the spiritual body. The spiritual body permeates the whole physical body with its sacred information, which acts intelligently for higher sacred states of consciousness.

24

Prayer Unifies All Humanity

Underlying the diversity of religion is a unified core that could be called spiritual religion.

—Elton Trueblood

I am thankful for my ERT seminar. Learning to pray aloud has changed my life. I discovered a powerful divine connection beyond anything I had experienced with silent prayer.

—Jody Kraner of Rootstown, Ohio

In the next chapter of this book you are going to learn to pray aloud. You are going to learn to vocally pray with others. Now, don't close this book! This chapter is designed to prepare you for the most powerful divine connection you have ever experienced!

Praying does similar things to what Emotion Release Therapy provides. It heals your hurts. It is intended to bring peace and unity among those with whom you pray.

The following chapter is intended to rid you of your cultural taboos about vocal prayer with others. It is intended to heal your shame, embarrassment, and fear about praying with others. It is intended to inspire you to become excited about praying.

Praying with others consistently links you with the most powerful divine connection you have ever experienced. I promise! So let us proceed with the prayer encounter with God.

It was my last Sunday as pastor of my church in Canfield, Ohio, and, as more than five hundred people left the sanctuary, they bid me farewell.

Paul, a 72-year-old widower, approached me, tears streamed down his cheeks, he warmly embraced me, and then he said, "Walter, I have been a member of this church all my life and you are the first pastor to teach me how to pray with others. It is such a joy! I pray with my children and grandchildren. I pray with my friends in the hospital. I pray for myself. I have never been closer to God. I feel like I have a connection with everyone in the world! Thank you! Thank you! Thank you!"

He had taken my course in oral prayer in which we, in small groups, learned to pray for each other's needs.

Do you know what really unites all the people on Earth? Not American rock music! Not satellite TV programs! The answer is prayer! The following statements reflect how all the people on Earth are united:

- The members of every religion pray. This amounts to some five billion people.

- Prayer is the primary means by which all people make daily firsthand contact with God.

- Prayers for healing take on universal characteristics that transcend religious differences.

- Human pain is universal, and praying for God to heal pain and disease is the main subject of the world's prayers.

- When people around the world have life-threatening or chronic medical conditions, they turn to persons of any religion for healing prayer.

- Firsthand contact with God results in a universal experience of awe, wonder, and oneness with the Creator and Sustainer.

- All religions share the common belief that God is the divine creator, revealer, sustainer, transformer, and healer.

- All religions believe that human beings are spiritual and are enhanced by contact with God.

- All religions believe in the afterlife.

- More than 90 percent of Americans pray, and about half of those who pray have no religious affiliation.

- Prayer is probably the most commonly accepted reality on Earth. Prayer is a unifying force between people.

I tell you this to overcome all the misleading stereotypes you may possess about praying with others. I tell you this to help you get over your reservations about sharing prayer with others.

During my ministry, I have prayed with more than ten thousand individuals and have had only one person refuse my prayers. Jews, Muslims, Hindus, Buddhists, agnostics, atheists, and Christians of many varieties have personally asked me to pray for healing.

If you are seeking common ground with someone, ask them if they pray. They may do a cultural double take at the unexpected question, but you are likely to find that prayer is a unifying factor between you and almost anyone else. When prayer is offered privately in an appropriate context, people universally welcome what it offers them.

As I was about to undergo major surgery at the Cleveland Clinic, a friend, a member of my church, visited me in my hospital room and prayed with me. The prayer was unexpected, but it was the most wonderful gift that Harry could have offered me at that time. Anxious before, I was now at peace and filled with joy. A prayer by you will be welcomed by anyone in the midst of a crisis!

Barriers to Praying with Others

The first barrier is that you have probably never prayed aloud with anyone. This is normal! Only about one percent of Americans have ever prayed aloud with their spouses for their needs. We have privatized our spiritual and prayer lives.

Everyone in your family probably prays. Every one of your friends probably prays. But you have likely never talked to any family member or friend about your prayer life. There is a strong cultural taboo about doing so.

So the first thing you have to do is get over your lifelong sense of shame about both talking about prayer and praying aloud with others. You can do this by releasing your inhibitions during ERT.

With no shame, pastors regularly pray aloud with others. Why shouldn't you? Identify your source of shame. Is it a fear of looking bad? A need to act respectably? Stage fright? Use Emotional Release Therapy to rid yourself of these hindering emotions.

Second, you probably have had little or no experience in praying aloud. So you feel unsure of yourself. You fear not being able to find the right words during a prayer with others.

Throughout this book, I have provided prayer models any time a prayer may need to be offered aloud. And in the next chapter I provide you with prayers for many occasions.

After praying several times with others, you will quickly be comfortable with praying aloud. You will discover that doing so is easy and rewarding for everyone involved.

Third, you may have a concern about religious differences between you and others with whom you may pray. I have discovered that if you refer to God as God, everyone is comfortable with that universal name for the Supreme Being. If you are a Christian praying with a non-Christian, you can be sensitive by not closing with Jesus or the Trinity. The prayer will be just as powerful.

Otherwise, prayers of concern have a universal language that is welcomed by everyone. Nothing expresses love and concern more powerfully than prayer. That person with whom you pray will feel a warm personal connection with you forever.

I often pray with strangers. In a hospital elevator, I see a person who is obviously in need of prayer. I'll say to the person, "Would you pray with me?" They always agree. I have prayed with strangers sitting on a park bench, strangers in waiting rooms, strangers at calling hours in a funeral home, and many, many other circumstances. I have never been refused. I don't introduce myself.

Fourth, is prayer a religious or a spiritual activity? A religion is a specific system of beliefs about God. Spiritual refers to personal contact with God, as through prayer. Obviously, prayer can be both or either.

I consider my prayers with others to be a spiritual activity for the therapeutic purpose of caring. Convincing an employer or a secular organization that your prayers are spiritual and not religious is all but impossible, but you can always try.

Praying aloud by yourself or with others is a more powerful spiritual experience than silent prayer. As one of my seminar graduates affirmed: "Learning to pray aloud has changed my life. I discovered a powerful divine connection beyond anything I had experienced with silent prayer."

Praying aloud with one person quadruples the power of God's presence. A Stanford University physicist has proven that the power of prayer is the square of the number of persons involved. One person praying is one prayer power. Two people praying is four prayer power. Three people praying is nine prayer power. Ten people praying is one hundred prayer power.

The average person releases two volts of healing energy in prayer. Two people praying together generate four volts of prayer energy. Ten people praying together generate one hundred volts of prayer power.

Taken in a scientific context, the brain operates on one-billionth of a volt. The heart operates on one-millionth of volt. Two people praying together produce four million more volts than the heart. No wonder prayer heals. It is very powerful!

This is a convincing reason to pray daily with the others in your household. Embrace or hold hands and pray aloud for one another's daily needs and for the needs of other vulnerable or hurting people.

When spouses do this at night while embracing as they lie in bed together, the results are astounding. It results in the rough edges of relationship disappearing, replaced by mutual peace and harmony. Remember the psalmist's wisdom, "Our hearts are restless until they find their peace in God." In the final chapter of this book, I offer prayers for spouses and families.

Daily praying aloud brings you an inner serenity and joy, a sense of vital purpose and actions designed to express caring, fairness, cooperation, and peace. Daily prayer permits God's presence to abide constantly within you and transform you. For me, prayer is a more profound spiritual experience than meditation. I think this is because prayer is more focused on practical needs.

Know the rules of praying with others:

1. Do not be condescending by asking to pray "for" someone. Treat them as equals by saying, "Will you pray with me?" or "Can we pray together?"

2. Always offer prayer in private. Private may be with more than one person. It involves every person with you when you pray.

3. Let your prayer be appropriate. Offer it in the context of your conversation and relationship.

4. Never try to manipulate people with prayer. Never use a prayer for advice-giving, as judgment upon another, or to ask God to somehow shape up the other person.

By praying aloud you become a priest. I define a priest as one who brings the power of God into the life of the world. Your prayers have this purpose and power. Rejoice in your priestly function of prayer!

25

United in Spoken Prayer

The energy of prayer destroys the chaos in and around you.

Prayer creates orderliness, purpose, and love in your life and the life around you.

Prayer provides an intuitive blueprint of God's purpose for you.

Prayer creates sacred clarity in your thoughts.

I encourage you to pray with someone else. But if this is not possible, I include in this chapter prayers for when you are alone.

Begin praying with family or friends. Suggest to them that you would like to pray daily with them. Mornings and evenings are the favorite times. Holding hands further empowers the experience.

If you live alone, you can also pray with family and friends over the phone.

Choose a prayer with which you are familiar from your religious tradition. For Christians, the Lord's Prayer is the most familiar. Write it out because in your nervousness you may forget a word.

If you are praying with other Christians, you can all pray the Lord's Prayer together.

At my suggestion, my parents in their seventies began praying the

Lord's Prayer together every night while embracing in bed before going to sleep. I didn't know that they were doing it until many months had passed. My dad finally shared, "Mom and I have been closer than ever as we've prayed the Lord's Prayer together at bedtime." As he said it, tears filled his eyes and trickled down his cheeks. They lived long enough to celebrate their sixty-fifth wedding anniversary.

When couples pray together while embracing before going to sleep, harmony and closeness abide. The same is true when parents and children pray together. Try it!

Don't feel selfish about praying for yourself. God has more than enough love to spare. Praying for yourself shows that you trust God.

Prayer is just asking God to bless you in various ways. So prayer language is not difficult. You are just unfamiliar with it. Going beyond the Lord's Prayer, here are some prayer models for you to begin with. Remember to hold hands.

Table Graces

- Come, Lord Jesus, be our guest. Let this food to us be blessed. God is great! God is good! Let us thank him for our food. Amen.

- God, thank you for making each of us special and important. Fill us with your love and help us to love and care for each other. Provide for our needs. May your peace fill our hearts and make us strong. We thank you for this food. May it nourish our bodies. Amen.

- God, the giver and sustainer of all life, remove our tiredness and fill us with life anew. We thank you for this food and those who have prepared it. Surround us in your presence and make us one with all whom we love. May your joy fill our hearts as we enjoy the remainder of this day. Amen.

- Thank you, God, for being with us today. Guide us and lead us in all we do. Bless our food and the hands that prepared it. Thank you. Amen.

- Thank you, God, for being with me today. Guide me and lead me in all I do. Bless this food and the hands that prepared it. Thank you. Amen.

A Bedtime Prayer for a Couple or a Couple with Minor Children

God, we thank you for this day. (You can list things you are thankful for.) Thank you for our love for each other.

Heal us. Restore every cell in our bodies and make us healthy and whole. Fill us with your love, joy, peace, and holiness.

Provide for our needs. Protect us from all harm.

We pray for _____ [names]. Heal them. Restore every cell in their bodies and make them healthy and whole. Fill them with your love, joy, peace, and holiness.

Provide us with a good night's sleep that we might awake refreshed. Guide and sustain us throughout tomorrow. Amen.

A Bedtime Prayer for a Couple with Grown Children

God, we thank you for this day. (You can list things you are thankful for.) We thank you for our love for each other.

We pray for our children and their families. Heal them. Restore every cell in their bodies and make them healthy and whole.

Fill them with your love, joy, peace, and holiness. Provide for their needs. Protect them from all harm.

We pray for _____ [names]. Heal them. Restore every cell in their bodies and make them healthy and whole. Fill them with your love, joy, peace, and holiness.

Heal us. Restore every cell in our bodies and make us healthy and whole. Fill us with your love, joy, peace, and holiness.

Provide us with a good night's sleep that we might awake refreshed. Guide and sustain us throughout tomorrow. Amen.

Prayer for a Person in Trouble

God, I pray for _____ [name] who is struggling. Keep him/her safe from all harm. Provide him/her with harmony in his/her life. Guide and lead him/her in this time of trouble. Heal him/her. Restore every cell in his/her body and make him/her healthy and whole. Fill him/her with your love, joy, peace, and holiness. Amen.

A Bedtime Prayer for a Single Person

God, I thank you for life. I ask you to bring me the fullness of life.

I pray for _____ [names]. Heal them. Restore every cell in their bodies and make them healthy and whole. Fill them with your love, joy, peace, and holiness.

I pray for myself. Heal me. Restore every cell in my body and make me healthy and whole. Fill me with your love, joy, peace, and holiness.

Provide me with a good night's sleep that I might awaken refreshed. Guide and sustain me throughout tomorrow. Amen.

Deepening Marital Love

God, thank you for joining us together in the rich bond of marriage. We remember the faith, hope, and love of our wedding day. We rejoice in our struggles and celebrations.

We keep before us the sacred wisdom: "Love is patient and kind. Love is not rude. Love does not insist on its own way. It is not irritable or resentful. Love rejoices in the right. Love bears all things, believes all things, hopes all things, and endures all things."

God, fill our souls with your love that we might always cherish and honor each other in gracious love. Amen.

About the Author

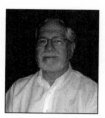

Walter Weston, born in Canton, Ohio, was for 30 years a United Methodist parish minister in Ohio. In 1989, he began a second career in holistic healthcare, focusing on spiritual healing.

In 1989, he participated as a healer with Ramesh Singh Chouhan, M.D., in the Chouhan-Weston Clinical Studies in India that scientifically verified a dozen theories involving the practice of prayers for healing.

In 1991, Walter Weston earned a doctor of ministry degree in prayer and healing research at the International College of Spiritual and Psychic Sciences, Montreal. His faculty advisor was Dr. Bernard Grad, a research biologist at McGill University and the father of healing research (he conducted more than two hundred healing studies).

Dr. Weston studied the scientific data, beliefs, theories, practice, and history of healing in the United States, other cultures, and the world's religions.

He has practiced healing with Christians, Jews, Hindus, Buddhists, Muslims, Native Americans, New Agers, agnostics, and atheists.

In 1994, his first book, *Pray Well: A Holistic Guide to Health and Renewal,* was self-published. It is a footnoted, well indexed, scientific encyclopedia on the scientific and rational understanding of healing.

In 1994, he developed Emotional Release Therapy, which offers dramatic healing of painful memories and destructive emotional states. He also developed the first scientific energy model for disease and spiritual healing.

In 1996, he went to Bangalore, India, to teach Emotional Release Therapy to pranic healers whose work was producing few healings. After their training, they reported that every person who used Emotional Release Therapy first was healed by pranic healing.

In 1998, Hampton Roads published three of Dr. Weston's books: *Healing Others: A Practical Guide, Healing Yourself: A Practical Guide,* and *How Prayer Heals: A Scientific Approach.*

In 2000, Dr. Weston spent a month in South Africa teaching Emotional Release Therapy to Zulu schoolteachers and social workers, so they could use it with millions of children orphaned by the AIDS epidemic.

He has taught more than 3,000 people in the United States, Canada, India, and South Africa how to practice Emotional Release Therapy.

Walter Weston is an author, seminar leader, healer, psychotherapist, and wellness counselor.

He can be reached at wweston@neo.rr.com or P.O. Box 618, Wadsworth, Ohio 44281. Visit his website at www.emotionalreleasetherapy.net. There you can order this book or a five-hour DVD produced by him, which leads you through Emotional Release Therapy.

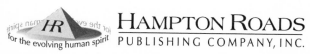
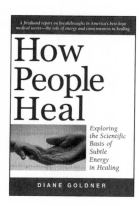
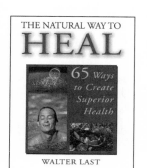

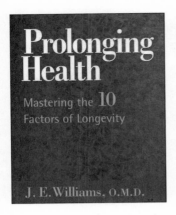

Prolonging Health
Mastering the 10 Factors of Longevity
J. E. Williams, O.M.D.

Based on the latest medical findings, Dr. Williams presents a practical, 10-point plan for anti-aging using the best of natural medicine. He shows how to strengthen your heart, revitalize your brain, rebalance your hormones, repair your DNA, and more. This definitive guide includes important information on "Aging and the Brain," along with advice for having an informed talk with your doctor.

Paperback • 464 pages
ISBN 1-57174-338-3 • $17.95

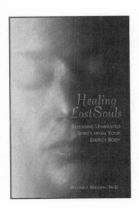

Healing Lost Souls
Releasing Unwanted Spirits from Your Energy Body
William J. Baldwin, Ph.D.

A therapist using the modern shamanistic techniques of Spirit Releasement, Past-Life Regression, and Soul-Mind Fragmentation therapy shows how physical and mental disease is often rooted in past-life trauma or entities attached to our energy fields. Not only does he tell you how to overcome these problems, but also how to boost your "spiritual immunity" to avoid them altogether.

Paperback • 336 pages
ISBN 1-57174-366-9 • $15.95

www.hrpub.com

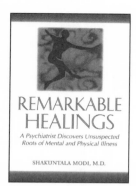

Remarkable Healings
A Psychiatrist Discovers Unsuspected Roots of Mental and Physical Illness
Shakuntala Modi, M.D.

Psychiatrist and hypnotherapist Modi presents startling evidence that attached spirits adversely affect our health and are the main cause of many illnesses. Modi gives you the signs of illness to look for as well as a "protection prayer" to help you heal.

Paperback • 632 pages
ISBN 1-57174-079-1 • $19.95

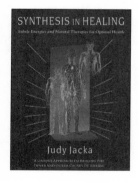

Synthesis in Healing
Judy Jacka, N.D.

Jacka explains the underlying factors of dozens of chronic conditions, from arthritis to insomnia to migraines and more. Then she explains how to reverse both the biological and spiritual causes with a combination of nutritional supplements, herbs, visualization, and meditative techniques.

Paperback • 344 pages
ISBN 1-57174-298-0 • $18.95

Hampton Roads Publishing Company

. . . for the evolving human spirit

HAMPTON ROADS PUBLISHING COMPANY publishes books on a
variety of subjects, including metaphysics, spirituality, health,
visionary fiction, and other related topics.

For a copy of our latest trade catalog, call toll-free,
800-766-8009, or send your name and address to:

HAMPTON ROADS PUBLISHING COMPANY, INC.
1125 STONEY RIDGE ROAD • CHARLOTTESVILLE, VA 22902
e-mail: hrpc@hrpub.com • www.hrpub.com